"In this compelling book, lauded card: Elefteriades recounts his most memoral who had "extraordinary" heart defects- more extraordinary courage. He explai: ment but also how caring for each patier a person. The book's engaging mix of sur it a fascinating study in the power of modern medicine and the tenacity of the human spirit."

—Denton Cooley, MD, Surgeon-in-Chief, Texas Heart Institute

"*Extraordinary Hearts* tells ten true-life tales of the extraordinary courage of ordinary people. Here are miracles and tragedies, faith and fate, and pure triumphs of the human spirit in the face of impending death. Dr. John Elefteriades's hands have touched the living hearts and saved the lives of more than five thousand men and women. His book will touch your heart and lift you up."

—Matthew Hughes, author of the *Tales of Henghis Hapthorn*

"*Extraordinary Hearts* is an extraordinary book. Dr. Elefteriades has brought the medical and surgical odysseys of ten of his patients to life. He is a most gifted surgeon but he is also a gripping weaver of true stories about cardiac patients and their operations. I must confess that after watching hundreds of cardiac operations I still consider an open-heart procedure to be a miracle. This book will engage those who practice medicine or surgery as well as the many others who are reading stories like this for the first time. I recommend this book to both groups wholeheartedly. The tales that these patients bring to these pages are unforgettable."

—Lawrence S. Cohen, MD, Ebenezer K. Hunt Professor of Medicine (Emeritus), Yale University School of Medicine

"This book provides a fascinating and seldom available insight into the reasoning, the concerns, and the technical considerations of a cardiothoracic surgeon as he goes about his work. In this case, there is even more: the stories reveal not only the complexity of the problems with which the surgeon must contend and the skills he uses to overcome them but, perhaps more importantly, the humanism of this particular surgeon, who is at the very pinnacle of his field."

—Jeffrey S. Borer, MD, Professor of Medicine, Cell Biology, Radiology, and Surgery; Chief, Division of Cardiovascular Medicine State University of New York, Downstate Medical Center, and SUNY Downstate College of Medicine; Director, The Howard Gilman Institute for Heart Valve Diseases and the Schiavone Cardiovascular Translational Research Institute

continued . . .

"*Extraordinary Hearts* by Dr. John A. Elefteriades takes the reader vividly into the cardiac surgery operating room, a world in which brilliant minds and good hearts of different people get interconnected. In this milieu, the reader is exposed to the bravery and courage of heart disease patients who put their lives in the hands of talented 'strangers' and the intense sacrifice that is required from the cardiac surgeon in these operations. Each of the ten stories in this book is a thriller in every sense of the word. These patients are being followed from the moment they are brought into the operating room, and until the surgery is over you cannot pause reading. By telling the story of every patient and introducing us to these incredible individuals, this fascinating book reveals the source of inspiration and strength that keeps the surgeon fighting relentlessly for the patients' lives and how the surgeon's own life is being enriched by each encounter."

—Asher Kimchi, MD, FACC, FAHA; Clinical Chief, Division of Cardiology, Cedars-Sinai Heart Institute, Los Angeles; Clinical Professor of Medicine, David Geffen School of Medicine at UCLA; Chairman, International Academy of Cardiology

"To be able to educate whilst drawing you into gripping tales of the power of the human spirit is no mean feat. Yet in this book Dr. Elefteriades has managed to do just that. I finished this book not just completely inspired by the stories in it, but also feeling like I'd been a part of Dr. Elefteriades's medical team! Through his eyes we are privileged to gain a unique and often hidden insight into the world of the operating theatre. Honest, touching, fascinating, empowering, and accessible."

—Sophie Robinson, producer, BBC Documentaries

"*Extraordinary Hearts* is a wonderful book, providing a unique peek into the mind of one of the United States' leading heart surgeons and the lives of those in his care. I've had the great privilege of seeing John Elefteriades at work in the operating room and I can tell you that these stories are as mesmerizing as his surgical craft."

—Kevin Fong, MD, host of BBC *Horizons*

"*Extraordinary Hearts* is a must-read for health-care providers and the public alike. Dr. Elefteriades's expertise and compassion shine through in every word. The stories are not just about illness and the miracles of modern medicine. They are about the unbelievable human spirit displayed by doctors and patients alike. Yes, readers will learn about heart health but, even more than that, they will be inspired by the strength, passion, and commitment shown by the doctors and the people they treat." —Carolyn Levering, president and CEO of The Marfan Foundation

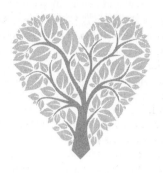

Extraordinary
HEARTS

A Journey of Cardiac Medicine
and the Human Spirit

John A. Elefteriades, MD

BERKLEY BOOKS, NEW YORK

THE BERKLEY PUBLISHING GROUP
Published by the Penguin Group
Penguin Group (USA) LLC
375 Hudson Street, New York, New York 10014

USA • Canada • UK • Ireland • Australia • New Zealand • India • South Africa • China

penguin.com

A Penguin Random House Company

This book is an original publication of The Berkley Publishing Group.

Copyright © 2014 by Dr. John A. Elefteriades.
Appendix illustration on page 264 previously appeared in *Scientific American*,
August 2005, Vol. 293, Issue 2.
Appendix illustrations copyright © John A. Elefteriades.
Penguin supports copyright. Copyright fuels creativity, encourages diverse voices,
promotes free speech, and creates a vibrant culture. Thank you for buying an authorized
edition of this book and for complying with copyright laws by not reproducing, scanning,
or distributing any part of it in any form without permission. You are supporting writers
and allowing Penguin to continue to publish books for every reader.

BERKLEY® is a registered trademark of Penguin Group (USA) LLC.
The "B" design is a trademark of Penguin Group (USA) LLC.

Library of Congress Cataloging-in-Publication Data

Elefteriades, John A., author.
Extraordinary hearts : a journey of cardiac medicine and the human spirit / John A. Elefteriades.
p. ; cm.
ISBN 978-0-425-27152-0
I. Title.
[DNLM: 1. Elefteriades, John A.   2. Cardiac Surgical Procedures—Personal Narratives.
3. Thoracic Surgery—Personal Narratives. WG 169]
RD598.35.C35
617.4'12—dc23
2013048633

PUBLISHING HISTORY
Berkley trade paperback edition / April 2014

PRINTED IN THE UNITED STATES OF AMERICA

10 9 8 7 6 5 4 3 2 1

Cover illustration © iStockphoto/Thinkstock.
Cover design by Judith Lagerman.
Interior text design by Tiffany Estreicher.

The publisher does not have any control over and does not assume
any responsibility for author or third-party websites or their content.

*Penguin is committed to publishing works of quality and integrity.
In that spirit, we are proud to offer this book to our readers;
however, the story, the experiences, and the words
are the author's alone.*

This book is dedicated to Dr. Denton Cooley,
heart pioneer and surgeon extraordinaire—without whose
personal courage, exceptional insight, and supreme technical
skills the dramatic surgical procedures described in this
text would never have been developed.

I wish to thank Adam Kane who, in reviewing a very early

ACKNOWLEDGMENTS

I wish first to acknowledge the special patients and their families who have allowed me to tell their stories in this book. Not only have they dealt with life-threatening—sometimes life-ending—cardiac situations, but they have had the strength of spirit that it takes to allow others to share in the intimate details of their health and lives. I am grateful to the patients and their families who have provided to me records and memorabilia, which have enhanced the preparation of this book.

I wish to acknowledge Ms. Marianne Tranquilli, our nurse specialist, who took care of each and every one of these patients together with me. She has known and bonded with them exceptionally strongly.

I wish to thank Adam Korn who, in reviewing a very early

version of this work, encouraged me to emphasize the impact of each case on me personally and emotionally.

A very special acknowledgment goes out to Ms. Karen Gantz, who, after hearing me give a talk about my career to my reunion class at Yale University, had the courage to investigate my written work and, ultimately, to nurture and represent *Extraordinary Hearts*. Karen is both a literary agent and a lawyer, combining skill in both arenas into a formidable array of talent for author representation.

I am profoundly grateful to Natalee Rosenstein at Berkley Books in Penguin Group. I am honored and privileged to have an editor of such stature and ability as a colleague for this book. Her guidance has been invaluable. I appreciate as well the able assistance of Robin Barletta at Penguin.

I express appreciation to my talented academic assistant, Carol Calini, for her able editorial assistance and to Dr. Bulat Ziganshin for his expert help with graphics.

Thanks go out as well to my wife, Peggy, book lover since birth, who has carefully and insightfully proofread the manuscript for this book.

I extend thanks to the talented medical illustrator Alex Baker, who has provided illuminating visuals for this, as well as many of my prior endeavors. Appreciation is expressed also to talented illustrator Robert Flewell for additional drawings.

Special thanks go out to Shireen Dunwoody of Dunwoody Communications, whose investigative reporting and coauthoring contributed immensely to the chapter on the drowned family.

CONTENTS

CONTENTS

PREFACE

I am going to tell you some stories, and special stories they are. I am a heart surgeon. In the practice of my specialty, it has been my privilege to meet (and care for) some extraordinary individuals. It is their stories that I will tell you in this volume.

Some are stories of courage. Some are stories of medical miracles. Some are stories of persistent shortcomings that exist even in modern-day medicine. You will hear of many patients who have done well, but also share in my despair for patients who have died, despite the best that medical science could offer.

It has been my privilege to care for more than ten thousand of my fellow human beings in my career. In this book I will tell you about ten specific individuals whom I have come to know in the process of caring for their hearts. I have chosen to tell you about the cases that have moved me the most, those that revealed to me the extraordinary characteristics—be they talent, intelligence, resolve, resilience, faith, courage, or altruism and humanitarianism—of our fellow men and women, often at their most desperate times.

Many of the specific cases I describe to you will represent dramatic examples of the miracles of modern medicine, and of cardiac surgery, in particular. In the course of hearing about these special people, you will learn about heart conditions and cardiac reparative procedures. But most of all, I hope you will share with me an appreciation for the wonderful breadth and depth of the human spirit—as I have seen it expressed in the context of the personal and familial challenges posed by critical cardiac illness.

I hope and anticipate that you will learn some medicine as the patient stories are told—but I hope you will learn this with pleasure and no pain, like the proverbial child's "pill in the apple-sauce." I hope that the medicine, surgery, and anatomy relative to each specific case will find their way naturally by osmosis into your consciousness without undue effort and without diminishing the stirrings of emotion that I also hope to create in your own heart.

So come with me now on a journey through the ever-evolving territory that is cardiac disease. Share with me the privilege of getting to know the "Extraordinary Hearts" to which I will introduce you. I mean "Extraordinary Hearts" in two ways. First, in the literal sense—that the heart organs of these individuals presented amazing anatomic and physiologic problems, for which modern surgery offers remarkable treatments and solutions. But even more so, I mean "Extraordinary Hearts" in the nonliteral sense—in which "heart" encompasses the core strength and characteristics of a human being.

These are stories about people at their best in the worst of times. I would like you to share with me an appreciation for the breadth of talent, the fortitude, the courage under adversity, and the invincible spirit of the extraordinary individuals whose stories I will tell you.

Knowing and caring for these very special patients has taught me a deep and abiding appreciation for the human spirit. I hope you will be moved as I have been.

NOTE TO THE READER

After telling you each of these remarkable patient stories, I will add a few paragraphs relating how each individual patient experience has enriched my life and helped me to grow as a person. I will put these comments about the very personal impact on me in italics, to make it easy to tell what sections constitute the patient story, and what sections relate to the personal impact that these cases had on me.

The Daily Life of a Cardiac Surgeon

As you read this book, you will receive an intimate exposure to the daily life of a cardiac surgeon—myself. You will see not the dramatized and glamorized lives to which you are exposed on TV and in movies, but the real life, with both its genuine ecstasies and its overwhelming agonies.

I go to work each weekday about 7 a.m., and I get home anywhere between 7 and 9 p.m. It may seem at face value like a long workday, but not if you see it in my context. During the seven years that I was a resident, I worked all the time. That was well before the implementation of governmental work hour restrictions, which were instigated by the well-publicized death of a patient in a prominent New York hospital—a death brought about, it is maintained, by an error made by an over-tired young resident. In my era, I was lucky if I got home for a day a week. We all lived on adrenaline: the fear of making a mistake kept us alert. So my current schedule, which allows me to go home each night, seems like a permanent vacation by comparison to my time as a resident.

On Saturday and Sunday mornings, I go in early for rounds, finishing in about an hour or so. I do not see working on weekends as any kind of imposition at all. Without the rush to get to the OR that we have on weekdays, the weekend rounds give me a chance to chat with the patients, to get to know them a bit better. I also have more time to teach the residents, without the regular weekday rush. These weekend rounds I find not onerous in the slightest. I am comfortable the rest of the weekend, just knowing that I have personally laid eyes on each recovering postoperative patient.

As you might imagine, the wives of the cardiac surgeons of my era literally ran our lives outside the hospital and also raised our families. The wives knew before they married us what they were getting into (many were nurses or other hospital personnel—where else would a surgeon meet a possible mate?), and they rose to the challenge. For years, I literally did not know where our bank was—or our pharmacy, grocery, or dry cleaner's, for that matter.

Despite the heavy professional burdens, we cardiac surgeons have traditionally cherished the time we did have with our children. I am proud never to have missed my daughter's cello concerts or even a single one of my son's wrestling matches. (No other dad, I am told, made it to every one over four years.) The lives of currently trained surgeons have much better balance, and newly minted cardiac surgeons participate more fully in their family lives. Seeing this new era, many of our wives (including my own) have become embittered and resentful of the obligatory sacrifice of their own professional lives to permit their husband's demanding surgical careers. This is often a source of conflict, as the life patterns of that era are now completed and irreversible.

I operate every weekday, and I have done so for the nearly three decades since I went into practice. I have performed well over five thousand heart operations, including three hundred and fifty heart transplants, two hundred artificial heart procedures, and many thousands of coronary bypass and aortic aneurysm operations.

Like other academic cardiac surgeons, I spend much of my off time working on papers or traveling to give lectures. I have lectured and/or operated in thirty-one foreign countries, on all continents except Antarctica.

For this book I have selected the cases of patients who have deeply affected my life—enriching my existence by virtue of my knowing and caring for them. There were many scores whose stories I could have told, but I have chosen to share with you my life-changing encounters with ten most special individuals. You will read in this book not only our triumphs, but also our failures to correct the ravages of cardiac disease.

I am honored to have you share in the stories and meet some "Extraordinary Hearts."

Chapter

1

Mrs. Solomon

MIRACLE IN ROOM 13

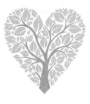 Miracles do not always announce themselves with choirs of angels. Sometimes a participant in a miracle does not even recognize that the extraordinary is happening. I had no idea whatsoever that a miracle was transpiring as I ministered, urgently, in the operating room, to a woman I later came to know as Emmy, who had just been critically wounded in that very operating room.

I had just sat down at my desk, with a Diet Coke and a yogurt, for the two-minute downtime that is my usual lunch period. My staff kindly allow me these few moments of peace before tossing me back into the constant stream of calls to patients, calls to physicians, new patient consultations, and assorted administrative crises that are all part of the working day for the chief of cardiothoracic surgery at Yale University School of Medicine. I do not have much time for myself during the working day, but for the next few minutes foremost on my personal agenda was getting a meager lunch.

My surgical team and I had done an aortic arch replacement that morning—one of the most technically demanding procedures in cardiac surgery. It had gone exceedingly well, and I was pleased with the outcome. Aortic surgery is our specialty at Yale University; we expect things to go right when we're operating, and we blame ourselves unmercifully if the patient does not do well, even in desperate cases where the odds are stacked against us. Still, it is always a good feeling when everything comes together and we can say, "That was a job well done."

I had just dipped a spoon into my blueberry yogurt when my secretary, Lorena, buzzed me from her desk outside my office door. "John," she said, "Dr. Stanhope needs you right away in Room 13."

Even before she had finished telling me what had happened, the adrenaline was flowing into my system. Lorena never, ever calls me by my first name. And when she added the words, "Their trochar went into the heart and the patient is bleeding to death," I already knew that the chances of this accident turning out well were hovering between slim and none. A trochar is a sharply pointed, hollow instrument that is used to insert tools into the body's chambers. It is an important part of the new breed of "noninvasive" procedures.

From my office to OR 13 was a distance of perhaps half a mile through Yale Medical's maze of interconnected buildings thrown up over the last century. I ran all the way, dodging people and gurneys, with my mind on one thing: A trochar wound to the heart would be messy, more like a battlefield injury from the time when men fought each other with swords and bayonets. The patient's chances of survival were minimal.

I reached the lockers near the operating room and quickly changed into my blue scrubs. There was no time to scrub myself sterile. I ran down the hallway and burst into OR 13, a room equipped for lung surgery. The scene I encountered was like something from a front-line dressing station in a war zone. No neatly arrayed surgical drapes, no carefully placed sterile towels and EKG pads, no soft-voiced instructions and polite responses from the staff. Instead, I saw that the drapes had been thrown aside—I could even see the table itself—and large patches of the patient's skin were exposed that had not even been painted with the red antibacterial solution we use to protect against infection.

I had to surmise what had happened, as there was desperate shouting all around, but no one was explaining what had transpired. As best I could tell, the surgical team had been performing a procedure on a small area of the patient's chest. The trochar had slipped and penetrated the heart. Now they had thrown aside the drapes so that they could use a saber saw to slice through the breastbone and get to the wounded organ before the patient bled to death.

The room had become crowded with doctors and nurses, most of whom had joined in when the accident occurred, their voices raised in a cacophony of orders and reports. I took a look at the monitors, seeing an unstable cardiac rhythm and only the vestiges of an arterial pulse. The chief anesthesiologist was surrounded by a squad of people who were pumping uncross-matched blood—the kind used only in absolute emergencies—and powerful tonic drugs designed to sustain a failing heart. As I entered, I heard the anesthesiologist call to the surgeons, "Come on, guys. Our hands aren't strong enough to pump the blood as fast as you're losing it."

There is no room for sentiment in an operating room, especially when things have gone suddenly, desperately, wrong. A surgeon has to summon up his inner "ice man" to assess the situation clearly and dispassionately. I did so as I shouldered through the mass of surgeons and assistants and muscled my way to the table. My immediate assessment was that this patient was surely going to die.

Dr. Emily Farkas, a first-class surgical resident, was doing her best to stitch closed an inch-long irregular tear in the heart's left ventricle, the organ's main pumping chamber. The heart was resisting her efforts. Its own beating, though feeble, was strong enough to tear the muscle further each time she engaged the needle. Opposite her was the distinguished, highly respected, and extremely talented Dr. David Stanhope, his eyes showing shock and dismay as he did his best to help her. His eyes were saying, "How did this happen? How did we fall so instantly into this bottomless pit?"

There was no time for explanations or professional courtesies. I slipped on a gown and surgical gloves proffered by the scrub nurse—sterility had gone by the board anyway and we would have to take our chances with infection—and said to Emily, "Let me in." She moved aside, and as I took her place, I saw a flash of relief in Dr. Stanhope's eyes.

The wounded heart had fibrillated, meaning that it had descended into the chaotic, ineffectual rhythm that is part of cardiac arrest. The anesthesiologist reported, "We are acidotic, pH 6.9. I have no rhythm or blood pressure. We're losing her. In fact, she's gone." The anesthesiologist, Dr. Jan Ehrenwerth, had decades of experience and was not one to mince his words.

In addition to all that, I could see, between rare organized heartbeats, that the patient's heart had been sucking air into the left ventricle through the open wound. That signified that the heart had certainly been sending bubbles into the bloodstream. When those bubbles reached the brain, they would block small arteries, cutting off oxygen. When the brain is denied oxygen for even a short time, neurons start to die. Even if we somehow managed to save this woman's life, we were all convinced that she would live that life with permanent brain damage.

Dr. David Stanhope had only recently joined us, to expand and improve our capabilities in lung surgery. He and I had never worked directly with each other before, but now we operated as smoothly as if we had stood together at this operating table a thousand times. It was clear that we had to get the patient connected to a heart-lung machine, which would generate a blood pressure, collect the shed blood, and provide circulation for the patient while her heart lay still. That was the only course that might permit us to render some sort of repair to the rent cardiac muscle. One of us massaged the heart as the other put in the stitches needed to attach the patient to the heart-lung machine, which was just now, upon my order, being hastily wheeled into the OR. The crowd parted to allow the bulky machine to take its place near the operating table. We inserted the arterial cannula— a medical term for a tube that can be installed in the body—into the aorta, and then placed the venous cannula into the right atrium. Valerie, our best cardiac scrub nurse, summoned from other duties, joined in at the table to replace the lung scrub nurse, who was not specifically trained for this amplified level of surgery. Valerie and I had worked together for two decades; I was very pleased to sense her presence, and now the rhythm of the operation improved.

While this was going on, there was time to catch up, and even time to observe some professional courtesies. Instead of requiring my more senior colleagues to relate how the devastating surgical accident had happened, I gave that task to the junior resident. In spurts of a few sentences, I got incomplete snippets of information from him.

He had been starting the procedure on his own. David Stanhope, the attending surgeon, had been finishing another procedure in the adjacent room. The junior resident had passed the trochar under the breastbone, aiming for the left chest cavity. The patient had two nodules in the left lung and the aim was to perform a biopsy noninvasively. The hollow trochar would allow first the insertion of a thoracoscope, a device with a lens and light source that would permit the surgeon to examine the nodules visually, and afterward the insertion of an instrument to remove and retrieve the nodules.

But then it had all gone wrong. Suddenly the patient's blood pressure had plummeted. The junior resident had called in David and Emily, who quickly determined that blood must be accumulating in the pericardium, the sac that surrounds the heart. That would put external pressure on the heart. That pressure would prevent the heart from taking in blood normally and pumping it out, resulting in a shock state. Emily and David had torn the drapes apart, opened the breastbone wide, and seen immediately that the thumb-width trochar had penetrated the left ventricle. They had begun trying to repair the large, irregular, stellate gash when I came in.

The patient was on the heart-lung machine now, her heart isolated from her body. I could now lift the heart for a careful examination. The tear was bad, very bad. The heart muscle, although strong as a pump, is too frail to hold stitches securely. The sutures Emily had placed earlier when the heart had been beating had all torn through the heart muscle, further enlarging and aggravating the hole. I could easily place two fingers in the wound.

But there was something we could do. Over ten years ago, a firebrand Brazilian heart surgeon named Randas Battista developed effective techniques for suturing friable heart muscle tissues, as part of a heart operation (bearing his name) that is no longer performed. But the suturing techniques Battista developed stayed in the consciousness of heart surgeons throughout the world. Now, in Yale OR 13, we applied those techniques to this dying patient. With the heart lying still, we placed wide bites of heavy suture across the hole in the left ventricle. We supplemented those with smaller bites at the precise site of the tear. Then we reinforced the stitches with Teflon felt, to keep the sutures from tearing through like a wire cutting through cheese. Finally, on top of the repair we placed some surgical tissue adhesive—the stuff we call "glue."

Yet all the time I was doing this, I knew the patient could not survive. We were just going through the motions, because I felt I had to support my embattled surgical colleagues as best I could. They would do the same for me if the roles were reversed. But we had to face the hard, cold facts: This patient had been without a blood pressure for too long, her blood acids had risen too high, the heart had been injured and handled too much, and even if by some miracle her heart could sustain a heartbeat, her brain would surely be dead from all the time she had lain on the table without blood pressure and oxygen flow. And even if she survived with inevitable brain damage, she was bound to succumb to infection. The operating field had not been sterile. Unsterilized equipment, such as EKG wires, had passed right over the gaping incision, giving the ubiquitous germs of our environment an open door to the heart and into the bloodstream.

Still, you do what you must. We finished our tenuous repair of the cardiac tear. We called for the "paddles." We gave a jolt of electricity to the heart muscle. The quivering fibrillation stopped. First one beat, then another, then a string of beats, then remarkably, a normal cardiac rhythm established itself. Of course, the heart was not pumping any blood. The heart-lung machine was still doing that.

Cautiously, we started "weaning" the patient off the heart-lung machine, transferring the burden of pumping blood from the machine to the traumatized and sutured heart. The heart willingly accepted the load. We saw nice "blips" on the monitor, each one representing a surge of blood through the arteries. *Damn*, I thought, *this heart wants to pump.*

How about the repair? Could it possibly hold? It is a standard principle of cardiac surgery that you inspect all the surgical sites before loading the heart and taking the patient off the heart-lung machine. In this case, the repair site was so precarious that I was afraid even to lift the heart to check it. The mere lifting, I feared, would stress the friable repair site enough to make it bleed. And this was the left ventricle that we were talking about. Bleeding from the left ventricle is a bad, bad thing. David and I tacitly agreed, without a word said, that we would not lift and check the repair. It was what it was. If it held, it held. There was nothing more we could do.

Amazingly, the heartbeats became stronger and stronger. The

anesthesiologist called out, "BP 70 over 40," not the 120 over 80 that we like to see, but beggars can't be choosers. A minute or two later, as Dr. Ehrenwerth administered cardiotonic agents by vein, he announced, "90 over 60." A few minutes later, we heard the magic triple-digit number "100 over 70." We were in a range adequate to support life. But could this improvement possibly be sustained?

Amazingly, the BP continued in a normal range. As far as we could tell, there was no massive ongoing bleeding from the ventricular repair site. I doubted the repair would hold securely for very long—perhaps a few minutes, I thought—but we were glad to take whatever forward progress we could get.

We washed out the chest cavity with antibiotic solution, and then we began to close up. The patient was, expectedly, rocky, with BP up and down, persistent acids in the bloodstream, and a continued need for transfusion (to replace the volumes that had been lost) and for agents to assist the blood to clot, now that we were off the heart-lung machine.

When we had closed the skin, we removed the disheveled vestiges of what had been the original surgical drapes. I saw a middle-aged woman, massively swollen from the fluid administration, cold to the touch from shock, and widely black and blue from the hastily created emergency opening of her chest.

I had done all I could. My office work was still piled on my desk and frustrated new outpatients were unhappily pacing the hall back at my office, waiting to be seen. They knew nothing of the drama that had made me late for their appointments. I left behind me a somber operating room. We were all surprised to have made it this far with the patient, but not a single one of us held out any hope for survival. The repair site could give way at any moment, leading to catastrophic internal hemorrhage and death. The blood pressure had been too low for too long. There was no way that the brain could withstand the effects of that low pressure. Besides certain brain damage, all the woman's other internal organs, including her liver, her kidneys, and her intestines, were not likely to recover from the advanced state of shock she experienced for such a long time. Her blood pressure was still wavering dangerously, requiring continued administration of blood, fluids, and the strongest available cardiotonic drugs.

And there was one other factor that deeply affected the mood in that OR. We all knew that the problem, the hole in the heart wall, was what we called "iatrogenic"—a Greek word meaning "doctor (*iatro*) caused (*genic*)." We had broken the first rule of another Greek—the ancient physician Hippocrates—whose ethical oath, having stood the test of centuries, requires that when we set out to heal, we first do no harm.

Back in my office, I dialed the phone to dictate my portion of the emergency cardiac procedure. It was then that I realized I did not even know the patient's name. In fact, I didn't know her precise age, either. While we were undraping, I had gotten some fragmentary basic information. She was about sixty years old. She had originally presented with cancer of the intestines. Her large intestine had been removed several years ago. Then she had developed cancer of the liver. The superb cancer surgeon,

Dr. Ronald Salem, had done a liver resection. Next, her abdominal lymph nodes had tested positive for tumor. The peritoneal fluid, which bathes the entire abdominal cavity, had also been positive for tumor cells.

These were extremely negative findings. Not much hope was offered. Still, under the direction of oncologist Dr. Barbara Burtness, the patient had undergone intensive, nonstop, three-drug chemotherapy for eighteen months. And then she had presented with the two small nodules in her lung. Today's operation was supposed to have seen their removal. The procedure had been described to her as minor, so her husband was not even in the hospital that day; he was out of state, at their daughter's house in Kentucky.

I finished my office hours. I did not stop by the Intensive Care Unit to check on the patient. Dr. Stanhope was her primary surgeon, and I had just been the emergency consultant. In fact, I doubted that she even made it to the ICU. She had been quite unstable, and the trip to ICU from the OR would constitute a survival challenge for such a patient. I strongly suspected she had died in the OR after I left, or during transfer to the ICU. That must be why no one had called to update me on her. I had fully expected to be kept in the loop, most likely to be informed of recurrent massive bleeding from the repair site, of continued shock and acidosis, or of the confirmation of brain damage, or most likely, death.

I went home at the end of the day. I had dinner with my wife, Peggy. I worked on my papers and scientific projects for an hour or two, exercised, watched a little TV, and went to bed. I did think it was a little peculiar that no one had called me about the patient with the cardiac injury. But I rationalized that any calls would be going to Dr. Stanhope. More likely, there were no calls to be made, because the patient had probably died shortly after I left, and no one saw any reason to disturb my evening with the inevitable bad news.

The next morning, I started my early rounds in the ICU, as per my routine. I was so certain the woman with the cardiac injury had died that I did not even think to ask about her. I always start my ICU visits at the back of the ward. I had seen my first patient and was in the hallway heading for my next patient when Nurse Barbara Blanco approached me. She said, "Mrs. Solomon wants to see you. She knows you."

"Who?" I said. I had no patient by that name.

The nurse said, "You know. Dr. Stanhope's patient."

"What?"

I was floored. How could it be? That patient, still alive? Impossible! And if by some incredible stretching of the odds she were alive, she would be, at the very best, extremely critically ill. On the ventilator, unable to speak. What was this nurse talking about?

Barbara took me by the arm and led me into a nearby room. There I found a middle-aged woman, sitting up in bed, smiling, looking extremely well, and having a light breakfast.

"Hi, John," she said. "Thank you for everything you did."

Who was this? Why was she calling me by my first name?

"It's Emmy, Emmy Solomon. I know I don't look my best, but take a close look and you will recognize me. They explained what happened. I am so lucky that you were available. Thank you for your skills and attention. God was watching over me. There was an angel hovering over me."

Little by little, I began to fit together the pieces of the puzzle. Of course, I knew the name "Emmy Solomon." She lived in my town. She had taught my kids in school. I had met her only once or twice, but I knew she was very close with my wife and children and that she was uniformly loved and admired in our community.

"I've been to your house," she added, further to convince me that I should know her.

"Hi, Emmy," I replied, still in a daze. I could not believe that this could possibly be the woman from yesterday. Her shock had resolved, the repair site had held firm, all her internal organs were working, she had been removed from the breathing machine, and obviously, from her bright expression and conversation, her brain was absolutely, totally fine. This situation would have fit any doctor's definition of unbelievable.

This was a miracle.

Emmy's next sentence reminded me of exactly why this woman was loved and admired by all who knew her. She said, "Thank you, John, for what you did, and please thank Dr. Stanhope and his team."

Remember, she had come in for a minor biopsy. What she got was a major iatrogenic emergency. Her chest had been sawed open to repair a doctor-caused tear in the main pumping chamber of her heart. She had been plunged into profound shock, put at risk of massive brain damage and death from systemic failure, and left with a hastily patched heart. She had barely survived. Anybody else would be looking through the Yellow Pages for malpractice lawyers. But not Emmy Solomon. What mattered to her was that she was still alive, and she was truly grateful to all her caregivers.

When I had been operating on her, I had had no idea that she was my children's teacher, and no thought that she might be an extraordinary individual. I had been in full "ice man" mode, concentrating on nothing but the job that my hands and brain were trained to do. Could I have been so cool, composed, and impartial if my feelings had been engaged, if I had known that I was operating on someone who was a part of my life and my family's?

I don't think so.

I said good-bye to Emmy Solomon, told her that I would check on her later, and left to return to my rounds. But as I visited my patients and noted how their recoveries were proceeding, I was still dealing with the overwhelming, reality-bending surprise I had found in Emmy's room. It was like a well filling up as all the things I knew about her came back to me. She was more than a member of our community; she was a legend. Not only was she known as a beloved teacher of our children, but she was revered for her self-sacrificing devotion to children all over the world. She had to retire when she took ill.

In terms of material possessions, Emmy and Steve Solomon never wanted or accumulated much for themselves. Yet they had started Renaissance International, a nonprofit organization that cared for homeless street children in Brazil. Our local papers had run several articles about their efforts in Brazil. Steve now lived in Brazil year-round, running the New Horizons Youth Ranch, an orphanage for abandoned children in a small town named Christianopolis, located in the Goiana region of Brazil, midway between São Paulo and Brasília. Some two hundred kids, from teenagers down to infants, had called the place home since it opened in 1991. During the summer school break, if Emmy could afford the plane fare, she would fly down to join her husband in their good works. The Solomons' own children, now grown adults, helped out there as well.

Steve had attended Yale in the Graduate Psychology Program and the Divinity School, before going out into the world to work as a teacher, counselor, and youth worker, ultimately finding his vocation as a full-time humanitarian. Renaissance International is dedicated to relieving the suffering of the two billion children worldwide who have been born into poverty. The foundation seeks first to provide for children's immediate needs: food, shelter, clothing, and medicine. As well, it aims to provide vocational, academic, and professional training and guidance, to give these kids a shot at a sustained better life. And all of this happens in an environment in which the children come to know Christ.

At the time of Emmy's operation, thirty boys lived at the New

Horizons Youth Ranch. They had been rescued from abusive families, degrading slums, brutal street gangs, and stunting poverty. The ranch fed, clothed, and sheltered these lost boys, embracing them as a family of brothers and offering them a haven of security and trust. Some of the street kids who had been raised at the orphanage had now grown into young men, able to lead and teach the younger boys. They showed the current residents how to work in the orchard and subsistence-gardening programs, while passing on other life skills.

Surely the key principle of Christianity, and many other world religions, is to treat others as we would like to be treated ourselves. Most of us, most of the time, pay only lip service to this Golden Rule. Emmy and her family had taken the commandment to heart. They had sacrificed everything in their own lives to dedicate themselves to the care of children in the direst need, children thousands of miles away whom they would never have needed to know about. Emmy Solomon had lived a life of truly selfless devotion to the least among us. I must tell you that, as I write these words now, tears well up in my eyes.

As the day wore on, David Stanhope, his residents, and I ran into one another around the hospital; and naturally, we discussed the Solomon case. The word we used was, of course, "miracle." But even as I spoke that overused word and heard it said by others, it was beginning to dawn on me that, this time, we were using the term in its actual, literal meaning. And as more time has gone by, my conviction has only grown deeper: what happened that day in OR 13 was nothing less than a miracle.

Frank J. Tipler, the famous physicist who writes popular books for the advanced lay public, defines a miracle as a striking event that seems to defy physical laws and suggests divine intervention. Emmy's case certainly qualifies by these criteria. By all the odds, by all the statistical likelihoods that govern medical diagnoses and care, *Emmy should not have survived.* The cardiac repair should *not* have held. Her internal organs should *not* have functioned. She should *not* have regained brain function. She certainly should *not* have been sitting up the next day, eating breakfast, and thanking us for what we did for her. I do not think that we, the patient care team, were the determining factor.

I think that Emmy's God and her angel watched over her because she and her family are devoted to their fellow human beings. The commandment is: *Thou shalt love thy neighbor as thyself.* I know of no one who more powerfully exemplifies that commandment than Emmy and Steve Solomon and their children. I truly believe that a miracle saved Emmy's life when anyone else would have died. And I think she, more than anyone I have ever known, deserved that miracle.

Emmy's wound healed perfectly, without infection, despite our dramatic violation of sterile technique during the emergency surgery. Another miracle.

And lest you think that Emmy's saintly attitude of the day after surgery waned with time, please be aware that two months later she underwent the lung biopsy that had been aborted that fateful day. And she insisted that only Dr. Stanhope perform the repeat lung biopsy procedure. She held no grudge, and she would hear of no one else to perform the procedure. She went out of her way to let him know that she trusted him and did not want him to blame himself for the way things had gone that near-fatal day in the OR.

The repeat biopsy procedure went smoothly. The two small nodules were indeed malignant, related to the original colon cancer. Emmy underwent another round of chemotherapy, which she tolerated well.

All of this happened six years ago. Emmy remains alive and well. She dreams of returning to the ranch in Brazil. "The children need me," she says.

After I had written the first draft of this chapter, my wife, Peggy, and I had dinner with Emmy. I asked her to read what I had written and tell me what she thought. She read the manuscript, making a number of factual corrections and (no surprise— she is ever the teacher) a good number of grammatical, spelling, and copyediting suggestions. She sent me a note afterward. Here is her response to reading the manuscript:

> . . . I was breathless reading it! It's pretty amazing writing when the main character is so caught up in the narration . . . (like I didn't know how it ended . . .). It's an amazing story and I truly had no idea just how dramatic the whole event was! As for the part about my role on this earth . . . well, let's just say that my halo is blinding me. . . .

I truly deserve no credit for what transpired. It was all Steve and the Holy Spirit leading him. My daughter and I didn't go to Brazil 'til he was about a year or two into it (I was a phobic flyer. . . another healing in my life) and my Mom, who was a bilateral amputee, lived with me every summer so I didn't go 'til after she was able to move into assisted living in NH. Dawn [their daughter] *was the one who gave her father twelve years of her life . . . she dropped out of college to go and didn't return to the US until ten years ago. Our son, Denis, was adopted from Brazil. He was one of the boys in the program and the only adoption that occurred. He helped out but he was only fifteen at the time. There's more that I would like to tell John and he can edit as he chooses but I certainly don't want to come off as an American Mother Teresa!!*

Then Emmy reminded me of the Swarovski crystal angel that we had given her as an end-of-school-year gift a long time ago. She wrote: *I saw him standing by my bed* [in the ICU]. *There are just too many "coincidences" in the story to not believe that all events were Divinely orchestrated!!*

She wanted to emphasize certain points. She reminded me that her name is not "Emmy" exactly, although I have spelled it that way in the text. Her full first name is Mary Elizabeth. That was a mouthful for a child, so early on in life she started going by "M.E." She forgave me for using "Emmy" in the text.

First, Emmy wanted it to be clear that she is not the selfless humanitarian in the family. That distinction belongs to her husband, Steve. He is the one who founded and has sustained the orphanage in Brazil. The ranch has been his labor of love, and she, Emmy, has simply helped out.

She and Steve had been typical youthful newlyweds, finding their way after college, when Steve read the Bible and found that his calling was to help others. He had served in Vietnam. Upon his return, he matriculated at the Yale Divinity School, where he earned his degree. He heard about an orphanage in Brazil that was in trouble; the pastor and his wife who ran it were ill. At that time, the dollar was up and the Brazilian *real* was down; so Steve was able to buy 150 acres of beautiful farmland for the orphanage. The New Horizons Youth Ranch was born.

In all of this, Emmy emphasized, she was simply the willing and committed accessory to her husband's philanthropy.

Second, Emmy wanted us to know that she feels she has not done anything special or out of the ordinary. She explained that God gave her a gift: *I was born to be a teacher. Throughout my life, I needed to give back by using this gift.* This, Emmy explained, led to her devotion and satisfaction in teaching fifth grade for her lifetime. Both my children passed through her class, learned from her, and felt her special love.

Emmy described her life as a "series of miracles." I was moved to hear this, because I believe that I was a participant in one of them. She explained that the themes of her life have been resilience, perseverance, hope, strength, positivity, and prayer. Her mission, she has always felt, has been to help others through her teaching. As to her miraculous survival, she said, "God is keeping me around until I get it right."

Penetrating Wounds of the Heart

Penetrating cardiac injuries have been known for centuries. In the *Iliad*, Homer describes the death of Sarpedon, one of the sons of Zeus, from a spear wound to the heart. The first successful surgical repair of a cardiac wound was achieved by Hehn, who in 1896 sutured closed a knife wound of the heart.*

Small knife wounds can sometimes seal themselves, even without surgery; the powerful heart muscle can contract around a small wound, sealing it off from bleeding.

Larger knife wounds produce cardiovascular collapse, as they fill the inelastic pericardium, or heart sac, with blood, causing a situation called "cardiac tamponade." In tamponade, the pressure of accumulated blood in the heart sac prevents the heart from filling, causing cardiovascular collapse and shock. Cardiac arrest ensues, unless immediate surgical care can be provided.

In contradistinction to knife wounds, bullet wounds produce large defects that cannot seal on their own. Immediate surgery is required.

The case described in this chapter involves a cardiac wound resembling a major bullet injury of the heart. As you see, however, this wound was incurred not in a street fight, but in an operating room. And the injuring agent was not a bullet, but an errant surgical instrument.

*O'Connor JO, Ditillo M, Scalea T. Penetrating Cardiac Injuries. JR Army Med Corps 2009;155:185-90.

Taking care of Emmy has had a profound effect on me. I have always considered myself a spiritual person (since my thirties, at least), but Emmy's case brought me into direct contact with the power of the spirit, although I was unaware of it at the time. When I look back on what happened in OR 13, I see no possibility that events could have unfolded as they did under any normal clinical paradigm. Emmy should not have come through. That she did, I believe, was because of who she is and how much she and her family have done for others.

Faced with that realization, I have to examine my own life. How much do I do selflessly for others? Sure, my work has directly helped thousands of people with sick hearts. And yes, as a young surgeon, I did volunteer for three months doing surgery at the Albert Schweitzer Hospital in Haiti, the poorest country in the Western Hemisphere.

But let me be honest. Cardiac surgery, for me, is always hand-to-hand combat with death. I don't always win, as you will see when I tell some of the other stories in this book. But I'm sure no medal-earning athlete experiences a deeper thrill of victory than I do when I face down human mortality across an operating table and deny the old specter his chill prize. But what if those selfish moments of triumph were taken out of the picture? Would I still be so eager to help others with my scalpels and needles?

As well, there is the financial reward. I have always been a Yale University employee, with much of the proceeds of my work going to support university activities and educational and research missions. But my career has provided my family and me with a comfortable living. Would I do what I do if the financial return was not good?

Emmy's case has made me question the depth of my own commitment to the mission of helping mankind without regard for oneself and one's own family. Would I, could I, ever give up my life to serve the street children in Brazil—those innocents thrust through no fault of their own into a living hell from which there is no escape?

Emmy, her husband, and her family have devoted themselves, totally and permanently, to the true love of our neighbor for which our God—be we Christian, Jew, or Muslim—says we must strive. Yet those who can do what Emmy has done are few. I have to say that, compared to Mary Elizabeth and Stephen Solomon, I fall far short of the goal. I believe that Emmy's survival against all odds reflects an abundantly deserved reward for her selfless devotion to others.

And I believe that the least I can do is to tell you about these extraordinary events, in the hope that you will be touched by her example, as I am.

Excerpted from Ruth Schenk, "Forsaken Kids: New Horizons Mission Rescues Abandoned Brazilian Children." The *Southeast Outlook*, May 25, 2000.

Maral's mother was a prostitute on the streets of Brasilia, Brazil, when she left her newborn baby boy at a city orphanage. Years later, in a *Pretty Woman* movie-script scenario, she married a wealthy man and went back to the orphanage to claim her son.

It seemed that Maral's dream of having a home and family had come true. However, on the way home, Maral's mother issued a threat.

"If you ever call me 'Mama,' you'll go back to the orphanage," she warned.

Maral's dream quickly turned into a nightmare more agonizing than anything he'd faced at the orphanage—more hurtful because he'd hoped for so much more.

In a disturbing pattern, everything that went wrong at the house was blamed on Maral. If a lightbulb burned out, Maral was punished. If a door didn't work properly, it was Maral's fault. Weary of accusations, within a week, he ran away.

The police arrested him on the streets. When released, he walked back to his mother's house, but the house was vacant. Every stick of furniture, piece of clothing, and personal memento was gone. Maral's mother and her husband had disappeared, leaving no forwarding address or message for her son.

Abandoned twice in his short life, Maral said that empty house barely echoed the giant hole in his heart.

Homeless once again, he joined the other 30 million children left to fend for themselves on the streets of Brazil. Children abandoned as casually as yesterday's trash . . .

"Young children last less than a year on the streets," said Solomon.

And in Brazil, death squads roam the streets at night, bounty hunters who kill children for a mere $50 each. According to *Dateline NBC*, most of the assassins are military police hired by shopkeepers who want to end the begging and stealing because it's bad for business.

"Many in Brazil believe that no one can change these children, that they cannot be redeemed," said Solomon. "But Jesus makes all the difference. These children are not garbage. They are precious. At New Horizons, kids are turned around by the love of Christ.... Street children have value and worth. They are incredible."

Maral joined other children at New Horizons. It was a whole new world for him where children learn for the first time that they have value and worth—that God loves them more than they could ever imagine . . .

The motto is: *Forget your past and embrace your future.*

Chapter 2

Dave Brubeck

CHICKEN WIRE

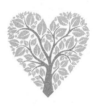I had just finished a heart valve replacement. I spoke to the family, giving them an ideal "early report," changed out of my scrubs, and walked over to my office, to check in with Gail, my "secretary"—as we were allowed to call our "assistants" in that pre–politically correct era. This was a couple decades ago. For some reason, Gail was excited about our new patient consult for that afternoon, who was expected shortly.

I stopped at my desk, picked up a few dollars in change from my drawer—my wallet was perpetually empty—and headed past Gail, out of the office suite that she and I shared. "I'm going to pick up a bite to eat, Gail," I said. "I'll be right back." She hated when I left, even momentarily, before she was able to deliver my

{ 27 }

urgent messages, seasoned liberally with her unique interpretation and social commentary, of course. Also, she had great judgment about medical issues, honed over years in her earlier post as ward secretary; she could tell from a phone call who was sick and needed prompt attention, and conversely, who was not and did not—all despite the fact that she had received no formal medical training whatsoever. Anyway, Gail was irritated, but my stomach called. I walked past her admonitions, into the hallway, in the direction of the cafeteria.

In the hallway, I passed a striking man walking in the opposite direction, toward my office. That must be "him," my mind subconsciously decided. He was tall, thin, and dressed in a blue one-piece jumpsuit. He had a huge shock of stark white hair, and a special intensity in his facial expression, plus a unique power and energy in his gait and his demeanor. He was a striking figure, instantly inspiring in his persona, albeit not aggressive or antagonistic in the slightest—radiating a sense that he was a man who knew who he was and what God had put him on this earth to do. All this I surmised with a glance, as we walked in opposite directions—he, I surmised, toward my office; myself, toward the café. He was accompanied by an austere, imposing, and somewhat stern-appearing woman; I presumed she was his wife. One could tell at a glance that she was the counterpart that made him whole. It was also immediately apparent, from their body language alone, that she watched out for the man by her side—and would continue to do so in respect to my professional interaction, assessment, and recommendations.

Of course, I was probably the only adult at Yale-New Haven Hospital who wouldn't have recognized him on sight. His face had been on the cover of *Time* and he had been profiled in *The New York Times*. He had composed and recorded albums that sold in the millions. He had been featured on network TV countless times. The State Department had sent him all over the world as an unofficial ambassador of American culture. If we designated people as "national treasures," the way the Japanese do, he would have been high on that list.

My only excuse for not recognizing Dave Brubeck on sight is that, although I have loved music all my life, God has not seen fit to bless me with even an ounce of musical talent. My high school glee club, though in desperate need of voices, asked me not to come around anymore. My tastes have always leaned toward popular music, especially with a beat that can drive my intense exercise sessions. I avoided classical music like the plague, and I never delved into jazz. Otherwise, I would have recognized Dave Brubeck and his wife, Iola, immediately.

Still, even if I did not recognize one of the leading artistes of America's premier musical art form, I knew I had just walked past someone special. I did not know then that I would have an opportunity to play a small part in extending a genius's career over another twenty-three years—and myself be profoundly and lastingly touched by the experience.

"You may recognize the name, John," Dr. Lawrence Cohen had said a week earlier when he had called to make the referral. "He is quite well known."

Dr. Lawrence Cohen was, and is, the "cardiologist's cardiologist," the one we consulted for spouses, parents, and when necessary, ourselves. His was the voice of ultimate authority in cardiology, the medical practice of heart care, in our region. Dr. Cohen was always calm and composed, unflappable really. He was also prone to understatement, as when he used the phrase "quite well known" to describe Mr. Brubeck. He could have said "one of the greatest musical talents of all time" and still been in the realm of a very conservative assessment.

Mr. Brubeck was then sixty-eight years old. He had been experiencing tightness in the chest during performances, accompanied by some shortness of breath. Dr. Cohen had suspected coronary artery disease, and a catheterization had confirmed it. All three of the vessels of the heart were involved, and Dr. Cohen requested that I perform an operation: a procedure called a coronary artery bypass graft, or CABG for short—and when doctors pronounce it, it comes out as "cabbage."

Arteriosclerosis can narrow a coronary artery, which is an artery on the surface of the heart that is responsible for providing blood flow to the heart. God designed our coronary arteries with plenty of built-in reserve capacity. The lumen, or central channel, of the artery needs to be restricted by at least 75 percent before blood flow is adversely affected.

In Mr. Brubeck's case, there was a blockage in each of the three main vessels of the heart. Just as traffic engineers build bypasses to route traffic around congested areas, we had to create other routes to get the blood flow to where it should reach. Accordingly, we needed to perform a three-way, or "triple," bypass. We needed to place a vein to two of the arteries, and an artery to the third. The artery used for this purpose is the so-called internal mammary artery, which we "borrow" from right inside the chest wall. The internal mammary artery takes its name from the fact that, in women, it supplies blood to the breast (the mammary gland). Grafts constructed with the mammary artery are especially durable; mammary grafts simply do not get arteriosclerosis, and they tend to last for the patient's entire life.

So on February 7, 1989, we took Dave Brubeck to the operating room. He was on the heart-lung machine for a total of two hours, with his heart "clamped" for fifty minutes. My assistant was our chief resident, Dr. Dimitris Nikas, who has since gone on to a distinguished career as an independent cardiac surgeon in his native Greece.

A heart surgeon cares about each and every patient, and during the operation, nothing else matters except that specific person and the one square foot of the world represented by the operating field. But there is an even deeper concentration when the patient is someone who has made a great contribution to humanity, and is likely to keep on contributing if he is able to walk out of the hospital whole and well again. So we all held our breath when the moment of truth came: We had put the bypasses in place and reconnected the heart to the body's circulatory system; now we applied the electric paddles. After a single shock, the heart started up beautifully and established a good rhythm. The heart beat strongly and regularly, and Mr. Brubeck came through the coronary artery bypass procedure with flying colors.

But then came the postoperative recovery phase, and some sleepless nights for his surgeon. Mr. Brubeck was generally doing very well until, a few days after the operation, he developed a rapid heart rate, a condition called atrial fibrillation. This is very common in the early days and weeks after open-heart surgery. Atrial fibrillation also becomes common with advancing age, affecting nearly 15 percent of the general population after age eighty. In Mr. Brubeck's case, the atrial fibrillation was worrisomely rapid, at about 170 beats per minute. And Mr. Brubeck tended to develop the atrial fibrillation late at night. Several nights in a row, I was in the hospital at 2 or 3 a.m. to treat this annoying rhythm disturbance.

To treat atrial fibrillation, we administer powerful medications to decrease the heart rate. Atrial fibrillation is common and rarely life-threatening after cardiac surgery, but the medications are dangerous—and I certainly didn't want anything going wrong. As well, back in 1989, we were very limited in terms of the drugs that were available for IV administration to treat atrial fibrillation; more advanced drugs were being used in Europe at that time but they had not yet been approved by the FDA for use in the United States. So each night, for several nights, we got Mr. Brubeck's rapid heart rate under control by administering some common, but powerful and potentially toxic, intravenous medications. I wore out the highway in the sixteen miles of I-95 between my house in Guilford and Yale-New Haven Hospital and lost a lot of sleep. All went well, however, and the atrial fibrillation became less frequent and easier to control.

On the fourth day after his operation, in the early evening, I went to see Mr. Brubeck. I wanted to be sure everything was in order before I went home. He was in the choice corner room, having been transferred out of intensive care the day before. I got the report from the nurse before going in to see him, and everything sounded in order. When I walked into his room, he was looking comfortable and well.

"How was your day, Mr. Brubeck?" I asked.

"Chicken wire" was his sole response.

I remember saying, "I beg your pardon," as I was not sure I had heard right. If I had, I certainly had no idea what those words meant. Many patients become confused after major surgery, and I was concerned that Mr. Brubeck was not making sense.

But he must have noticed the furrow on my brow, because he said, "You don't have any idea what that means—'chicken wire'—do you?"

"No, sir," I answered.

"Doctor, you don't know much about music, do you?"

As long as I was being honest, I thought I might as well admit that, too.

He explained the expression to me. When he and his band were starting out, the venues they played were not always choice establishments. "Some of them were just dives." And when they were playing for the kind of people who frequented "just dives," and those people didn't care for what they were hearing, the audiences would let the musicians know that their efforts were not being well received. They would communicate this displeasure by throwing things at the musicians: food, bottles, plates, and other assorted missiles, all of which could do some real damage. So management would put up a fence made of chicken wire between the bandstand and the patrons.

"Any up-and-coming band knows it helps to have the chicken wire up, to protect yourself and your instruments."

Mr. Brubeck was telling me he hadn't had a great day. His incision had hurt. He had had to go down for a chest x-ray. He didn't like swallowing the big potassium pill that patients needed to counteract their diuretics. And he had had another brief bout of atrial fibrillation, treated by the floor team. So, he was explaining, that all added up to a "chicken wire day."

But he was feeling well now.

I can remember the encounter as if it were yesterday. By that time, I knew I was in the presence of greatness, and to have Mr. Brubeck explain to me the expression "chicken wire" was truly a precious moment that I've enjoyed telling other people about— just as I am telling you now. And who would have expected that the great Dave Brubeck would ever have needed to play behind chicken wire?

Mr. Brubeck went on to do well—so well that I was able to leave several days later for a lecture trip to Japan. Dr. Cohen was to keep an eye on our special patient; Mr. Brubeck could not possibly be in better hands. In Japan, I was scheduled to do some lecturing and surgical demonstrations—all arranged many months in advance. I took my family with me, and we stopped overnight in Hawaii, to break up the long flight. We had never been there before. I was having breakfast on the hotel veranda, reading the local newspaper, when I saw a small article at the bottom of the front page. My heart surgeon's heart skipped a beat. BRUBECK UNDERGOES HEART SURGERY, the headline read. My heartbeat settled down when I read on and realized that the paper was reporting on the operation I had already performed, and that everything was fine: the patient had gone home in good condition. I exhaled a big sigh. Every cardiac surgeon has had the experience of unexpectedly reading or learning bad news about a patient. Fortunately, the newspaper that morning indicated that all was well with Mr. Brubeck. This was the first time—it was early in my career—that I read about a famous patient of mine in the newspaper. Thank God, all was well.

The coronary artery bypass operation is a truly extraordinary procedure—delicate, precise, effective, and extremely durable. It is now twenty-three years since Mr. Brubeck's operation, and he has never required any other procedure for his heart or his coronary arteries. The angioplasties that have become so popular in the present era—in which an artery is stretched by inflating a balloon inside the vessel and then a metal mesh tube called a stent installed to keep the passage open—cannot deliver the durability of a coronary bypass procedure.

Mr. Brubeck has distinguished himself extraordinarily as a true musical genius. His is a gift from God, honed with effort and love.

What amazes me most about Mr. Brubeck is how he remains down-to-earth and humble despite his extraordinary talent and accomplishments. He is polite and respectful to all, in daily life as well as onstage.

As I am writing the first draft of this chapter, I am watching Mr. Brubeck being honored at the Kennedy Center. It is December 29, 2009, and it also happens to be Mr. Brubeck's eighty-ninth birthday. Accolade after well-deserved superlative accolade is bestowed on Mr. Brubeck. He is being recognized for a lifetime of innovative achievement: He was a dominant force in increasing the popularity of progressive jazz. His contributions included the use of unique and varied time signatures—even 7/4 and 13/4 time—intensely complex rhythms, varied tonalities, and exceptional meters. Besides being a virtuoso piano player, he composed everything from oratorios to cantatas to Broadway musicals, and even the score for an animated CBS-TV series, *This Is America, Charlie Brown,* featuring the characters from Charles Schulz's *Peanuts.* His discography lists one hundred and seventeen albums.

At the Kennedy Center gala, a medley of Mr. Brubeck's music was performed by an ad hoc tribute band—the "Brubeck All-Star Jazz Quintet"—composed of bassist Christian McBride, pianist Bill Charlap, trumpeter Jon Faddis, drummer Bill Stewart, and saxophonist Miguel Zenon. They smoothly segued through the composer's iconic favorites, including "Unsquare Dance," "The Duke," "In Your Own Sweet Way," and the show stoppers "Take Five" and "Blue Rondo a La Turk."

But it was clear from the expression on Mr. Brubeck's face that the best part of the evening was when his four sons—all accomplished musicians in their own right—came onstage to perform selections from his works. When the show was being put together, Mr. Brubeck had asked the organizers if his sons would be able to play at the event. He was told it wouldn't be possible. That was because they wanted it to be a surprise. They swore the whole family to secrecy. And a surprise it was; that was most evident from Mr. Brubeck's expression when his sons came out. The result was one of the most poignant, beautiful moments I've ever witnessed, a great man beaming, with tears in his eyes, bursting with pride in his sons. Mr. Brubeck's four sons are playing his best-known tunes during the Kennedy Center tribute. Mr. Brubeck literally beams with pride. Such is the nature of the man—he himself has legendary talent, yet during the Kennedy Center proceedings, his greatest happiness comes not when he is praised, but when his children perform.

Chances are his thoughts go to his own mother, who trained him in music. Dave played piano by the age of four, and he was performing by fourteen. I can imagine his own mother's extraordinary pride and glee watching and hearing him play at those young ages; she must have sensed a superhuman talent.

His mother, as we have seen, was musically gifted and taught Dave the basics of the piano, but he didn't learn to read music, pleading poor eyesight. When the time came to leave home for college, being a cattleman's son, he opted for veterinary science at the College of the Pacific in Stockton. But his zoology professor soon realized that Dave's mind was not engaged and told him to switch to the music conservatory. He caught fire there with several of the faculty, except for one professor who wanted to expel him because he still couldn't read the notes. But his other teachers stood up for him, arguing that his grasp of counterpoint and harmony more than made up for the inability to read music. He did have to promise the school, though, that he would never try to teach piano.

The coronary bypass procedure added thousands upon thousands of days to Mr. Brubeck's life. He used those days to put music into the world. He toured constantly, playing all over the United States and in Europe, in virtually every part of the world except China. Playing the piano as a virtuoso is hard work; it demands tremendous energy and stamina. When I used to read about Mr. Brubeck striking the keys in some far-off venue, I allowed myself a certain satisfaction in a job well done: those three bypass grafts were providing enough blood flow to supply his heart during those animated, taxing performances.

Mr. Brubeck was a dominant force in achieving the popularity of jazz. He is known for brilliant contributions characterized by unique and varied time signatures, complex rhythms, varied tonalities, and exceptional meters. Mr. Brubeck also composed for orchestras and Broadway shows, including the highly successful *Mr. Broadway*. The Library of Congress characterized Mr. Brubeck as a "Living Legend." He has recorded 142 albums, many still actively produced and prized.

As I watch the ceremony at the Kennedy Center, jazz great Herbie Hancock takes the stage, to laud Brubeck and his accomplishments, citing Brubeck's album *Time Out* as the key musical inspiration for his own career.

Says Hancock: "When I first heard Dave Brubeck, that was the beginning of my long-term relationship with jazz. I had been playing classical piano since I was seven. When I was a teenager, I started listening to and playing jazz. When *Time Out* was released, it was a whole different spin on the jazz I'd been used to. Who could have imagined that this completely new music could be such a hit? This was 1959."

Anne Gerhart of *The Washington Post* vividly and eloquently captures the essence of the living legend Dave Brubeck by giving us a glimpse into his past. She explains that Mr. Brubeck's complex rhythm syncopations take their origins in part from the primitive beats of Africa. She goes on to give insight into the man from his early experiences:

It was his musically gifted mother who taught David, Howard and Henry, also musicians, to play piano, and it was she who insisted that David go to the College (now University) of the Pacific, and, once there, worried he was becoming a hermit. Take a girl to a dance, she said. Brubeck asked his roommate which girl was the brightest, and then he sent the roommate to approach Iola Whitlock. After some dancing, recounts Russell Gloyd, a conductor and former trumpet player who is Brubeck's longtime manager, David suggested they just talk. After three hours, they had decided to get married.

Profit Motive in Determining Choice of Cardiac Procedure

It must be difficult for patients and their families to choose between the options available for coronary artery disease (blockage of the arteries that feed blood to the heart muscle). This disease usually becomes manifest via angina pains or an actual heart attack.

Angioplasty, in which the coronary artery is stretched and then stented with a fine metal mesh, has become extremely popular. This procedure is done with a catheter, without an incision. The hospitalization is usually very short—two to three days. The procedure usually works well and is fairly durable—one can understand how the angioplasty procedure has become popular. However, over years, most patients need additional stenting, sometimes many times. We have seen up to ten or twelve stents placed in a single patient. Also, some heart muscle damage may accrue with repeated stent procedures.

The alternative is the well-known coronary bypass procedure, an open surgical procedure that requires an incision and four to five days in the hospital. Many studies have shown superiority of the bypass operation for patients with extensive coronary disease and demonstrated its unparalleled durability.

The decision regarding angioplasty versus surgery is very often determined by so-called "referral bias." The patient usually sees a cardiologist, a medical doctor, first. The cardiologist naturally believes in the angioplasty techniques that he practices and in which he has great expertise. Also, it is angioplasties that put food on his family's table. No doctor, like any other human, is immune to such influences. So the patient often does not get to see a surgeon for potential coronary bypass until late in his course, often after many angioplasty procedures.

We surgeons, of course, have our own biases—and it is the coronary bypass procedure that puts food on our tables.

This debate will continue for some time. As economic constraints increasingly impact the practice of medicine, regulatory agencies may impose incentives toward the more durable, cheaper (in the long run) coronary bypass procedure.

In any case—this debate aside—in the case of the great Mr. Brubeck, you see vivid evidence of the extraordinary effectiveness and durability of the coronary bypass procedure. One bypass procedure stood Mr. Brubeck very well for decades of life. He never needed any adjunctive later procedures—not even a single heart catheterization—as his bypass grafts pumped on and on, year after year, as he entertained and enriched the lives of millions.

Please keep one additional point in mind. If you or a family member are facing cardiac intervention, you may be told that surgery involves "cracking your chest." As a matter of fact, despite this derogatory choice of words, the breastbone incision is remarkably comfortable. Many of our patients do not even request or require any pain medication during recovery. Do not let the incision itself impact your decision unduly. Consider the long-term benefits rather than the short-term investments in your safety and well-being.

Note: Since this chapter was first written, Mr. Dave Brubeck passed away, on December 15, 2012, at the age of ninety-one.

As I am watching the Kennedy Center show, and the camera sweeps toward him, Mr. Brubeck is beaming a smile to the world as he waves to the crowd and the camera. It seems to me that this is a smile of satisfaction—with his career and his life—yet a fully humble smile. The applause of the audience is overwhelming. A tear starts to form in the corner of Mr. Brubeck's eye. I interpret that tear as his gratitude that God has given him the skills to entertain the world and to move the emotions of his fellow human beings. This man simply does not have an arrogant or supercilious bone in his body. His smile is one of gratitude, not self-congratulation.

As this chapter is being written, I have recently received Dr. Cohen's latest medical report on Mr. Brubeck. His heart continues fine, at the age of eighty-nine. Says Dr. Cohen, "He has passed his eighty-ninth birthday and is still quite active [with his concert tours]. I think he has finally cut back a bit, but there is always a tension between his creativity, concerts, and traveling, with the downside of the fatigue that comes with that type of program." Performing is Mr. Brubeck's life, and he continues to bless the world through his live concerts. (It makes me wonder about myself—specifically whether I will ever be able to stop what I do and love—operating on people's hearts. Surgery is a drug, and I am certainly addicted.) Amazingly, and gratefully, Mr. Brubeck has new CDs and shows in preparation—many years' worth, in fact.

I anticipate that hundreds of years from now, mankind will still be listening to and moved by the music of Mr. Dave Brubeck. I am confident that the sweet purity of the Dave Brubeck Quartet playing "Take Five" will make people close their eyes, smile, and tap their fingers. I hope that the knowledge of his special humanity and his humility continues into those times.

Then Brubeck went off to World War II, a sharpshooter who could play piano at the front. On D-Day, one of the many friends who died in the war was shot in the harness of his parachute as he floated to earth. Young Brubeck's anger and anguish deepened into faith and gratitude and an obdurate optimism that has driven him forward, a humanist, ever since.

"When that is what you experience as a young man," says Brubeck, "you tend to greet each day ever after happy to have awoken."

He always has known that music must be imperative for humans, because they create it. One night in a hospital bed 20 years ago, he was reflecting on the heart, his own, scheduled to be opened up to the surgeon's knife the next morning. He was composing, as usual: "Psalm 30," which he then dedicated to the cardiologist. He concluded that all rhythm begins, literally, with the heart—"pa-DUM, pa-DUM," he taps on his knee—its pacing changes, from emotion and duress, across climes and continents, perhaps accounting for the ethnomusical variations across the world.

"*It is the very first sound a baby hears,*" Brubeck notes, "*and the very last sound the body makes before it expires.*"

How has taking care of Mr. Brubeck influenced me and enhanced my life? Immeasurably. I feel that I have stood next to greatness. I have been exposed to the truly extraordinary combination, in one individual, of greatness housed side by side with genuine humility. I have seen and experienced firsthand Mr. Brubeck's living specifically for the purpose of improving the lives of mankind—through music. Mr. Brubeck, in my mind, represents an ideal of human character toward which we would all be well served to strive.

Chapter

3

Mr. Oliva

"THEY ARE BOMBING COLUMBIA
AND NYU . . ."

 We had just cut out the patient's aorta, the largest artery of the body. The aorta is the vessel that
takes oxygen-rich blood from the heart's left
ventricle and sends it out to the rest of the body.
The patient had presented with a large ascending aortic aneurysm: that means that the aorta had stretched and enlarged. The
deformation went all the way down to the heart itself, and all the
way up into the bend that we call the aortic arch. My surgical
team and I had hours and hours of work ahead of us.

Our patient was a forty-seven-year-old gentleman. Three days
previously, he had presented to an outside hospital with chest and
back pain and shortness of breath. His echocardiogram and CT
scans showed a number of pertinent findings.

First, he had a huge aneurysm of the ascending aorta; a normal aorta is about 3.5 centimeters in diameter—and his was 11 centimeters. Second, his aortic valve was leaking wide-open; it was as if his poor heart was functioning with no aortic valve.

The aortic valve is the main outflow valve of the heart. Can you imagine any mechanical pump—say a fuel pump or a water pump—working without a competent outflow valve? The work of the pump without such a valve is overwhelming, as the fluid that is pumped forward comes right back. The pump—or in Mr. Oliva's case, the poor heart—is overwhelmed by the excess workload.

Hence, Mr. Oliva's third problem: Because the organ was being strained to its limit by the leaking valve, his heart function was very, very weak. The "ejection fraction" measures the pumping strength of the heart. Normal is 60 percent, representing the fraction of blood in the heart that is propelled forward with each heartbeat. Mr. Oliva's ejection fraction was only 20 percent—or one-third of normal. No wonder he couldn't breathe. If the ejection fraction were any lower, he might not be alive.

As if those problems were not enough, the remainder of his aorta—the "good part," so to speak—was also distended by aneurysm disease, although not yet so massively enlarged as the parts that needed to be removed. But with his whole aorta dilated, the risk level in the operation we planned to perform was even greater.

And as if that were not enough, there was still more trouble. The backup of blood due to the malfunctioning aortic valve had affected the liver (too much back pressure), so that that organ was also dysfunctional. A malfunctioning liver makes it very difficult to survive cardiac surgery. And further complicating matters, the malfunctioning liver was not making adequate coagulation (clotting) factors, so that Mr. Oliva's blood was too thin. Thin blood is the last thing the surgeon wants to see before major cardiac and aortic surgery, because the blood needs to be thick enough so as not to leak through surgical suture lines.

This case was going to be an extraordinary clinical challenge, no doubt about it—with a high likelihood of the patient's not surviving.

We got to know Mr. Oliva hurriedly in the hours after his urgent transfer to Yale for specialized aortic care. He was a pleasant, somewhat simple man, who trusted completely in our team to provide his care. He worked as a printer's helper. He had been born and raised in the working-class town of Derby, Connecticut. He was heavily involved in the Boy Scouts of America, first as a Scout, then as a Den Leader, and ultimately as an adult Scoutmaster. Mr. Oliva had an abiding concern for nature and the environment. And he trusted completely that we would look after him.

We let Mr. Oliva know that his cardiac situation was serious, and we explained the general nature of his cardiac problems. We described the surgical approach and risks involved. But by his nature, Mr. Oliva was trusting and did not want to know many details. This is in contradistinction to so many of our patients, who have read extensively on the Internet and come armed with dozens of detailed questions. (Before the iPad era, the lists of questions were on paper and we could tell at a glance how many we would be asked. Now that patients bring along portable data devices, we never know how long a session will last until they work their way right down the electronic list.)

For all the difficulties his case presented, Mr. Oliva was a pleasure to deal with in every way. He showed remarkable courage in the face of an adversity that he may not have comprehended in detail but certainly understood in every sense that mattered.

After his arrival at Yale, we brought Mr. Oliva promptly to the OR, fearing that his massively enlarged aorta would rupture or that his straining heart would simply give up and stop beating. Pain is a terrible harbinger in patients with aortic aneurysms, because pain portends impending rupture. Mr. Oliva had just such pain. He also had advanced shortness of breath, reflecting cardiac failure, another indicator of potential impending cardiac arrest.

In light of all of these concerns, we were worried that Mr. Oliva might not survive if he was left to wait for his place in line on my operating schedule. Sometimes, in urgent situations like this, we need to disappoint one patient in order to safeguard another.

We now brought Mr. Oliva to the operating room in place of another patient. We hate to "bump" a patient in this way, because we recognize that people facing major surgery have had to prepare themselves mentally and physically, and it is hard for them to "stand down" just when they think the moment has finally come. But when necessary, in life-threatening situations, we have to ask patients to put another's need ahead of their own.

Accordingly, we brought Mr. Oliva to the operating room early in the morning. He was safely put to sleep by Dr. Bing Zhu, one of our most talented cardiac anesthetists, who had come to Yale from China as an anesthesia fellow; he did so well that he was asked to stay on as an attending physician. That was our first hurdle passed: in a patient so severely jeopardized, by a constellation of cardiac conditions, just putting Mr. Oliva to sleep was dangerous in and of itself.

With Mr. Oliva safely anesthetized, we commenced the operation. We knew the risk involved in the surgery would be very high. The aneurysm was huge. The operation had to be extended all the way toward the heart, right down to where the aorta joined the cardiac muscle itself. At the upper end, the operation had to be extended under the so-called aortic arch, the arc-like bend of the aorta at the top of the chest, which gives the vessel its "candy cane" shape. All of this would need to be done in the face of a failing, stretched heart muscle.

We split the breastbone vertically with a saw. The aneurysm was enormous, its sheer size displacing all the other structures. The heart itself was pushed down and to the left. The branches of the aortic arch to the head and arms had been pushed aside by the ballooning aorta.

We hooked up the patient to the heart-lung machine that would circulate and oxygenate Mr. Oliva's blood for him after we stopped his heart. The aneurysm was so large and extensive that we could not place the machine's arterial cannula (the tube that brings fresh blood to the patient) where we normally would, in the chest. Rather, we attached it to the large femoral artery in the groin. Then we started the heart-lung machine, so that we could stop the heart and freely operate on that organ and the diseased aorta. From now until we finished the operation, the machine would take over the function of Mr. Oliva's heart and lungs. Though he wasn't breathing and his heart wasn't beating, he could stay alive on the heart-lung machine for several hours, if necessary.

We stilled the heart then disconnected the aorta from the heart muscle. We selected a prefabricated graft that carried a valve inside it; the graft would let us replace the aorta and the valve at the same time. We sutured this composite graft onto the heart at the place where the massively enlarged aorta had been cut away. This is a serious and delicate operation, made more complicated by the need to reattach as "buttons" the two main coronary arteries, the important small vessels that supply blood to the heart muscle itself. Objective graders have classified this particular operation as the highest acuity of all adult cardiac surgical procedures.

While this was going on, the heart-lung machine had been deep-cooling the patient. The machine contains a heat exchanger, similar to a heating-cooling unit that you might use to warm or cool a room. As his blood passed through the machine, Mr. Oliva's body temperature was lowered so that his metabolic rate—

the rate at which biochemical activity in the cells occurs—fell dramatically. He now entered into a state known as deep hypothermic circulatory arrest (DHCA), or "the deep freeze" in medical slang. His tissues were not actually frozen, just deeply chilled. We disconnected him from the heart-lung machine, which meant he had no blood flow at all. His blood pressure was zero. His pulse rate was zero. His breathing rate was zero. He had no brain waves. For all intents and purposes, he was dead.

Now why did we need to cool the patient and stop circulation? That is necessary in order to work on the branches of the aorta at the top of the "candy cane." Stopping circulation permits work on the top of the aorta and the branches to the brain and arms in a bloodless field with excellent exposure.

The DHCA, suspended-animation technique is one of our specialties at Yale. We have thoroughly studied brain function in patients who have been exposed to this technique and have found that cognitive function is very fully preserved. In all my experience in medicine, I can't think of a more extraordinary technique. It goes against common sense, but it is a simply remarkable fact that the deeply cooled human brain can withstand forty-five to sixty minutes without any blood flow at all. The rewarmed patient awakens later in the day with full cognitive capacities and all reflexes, memories, and learned facts and skills fully intact. But while the patient is in the deep freeze, the surgical team must work fast. If the delicate and challenging reconstruction of the brain arteries is not completed within that narrow window of sixty minutes, the result can be disaster.

Mr. Oliva had to be put into the deep freeze so that we could work on the branches of the aorta at the top of the "candy cane"— the blood vessels that supply the brain. This most delicate stage of the operation cannot be performed while blood is still circulating in the aorta. So when we had finished placing the graft at the lower end of the diseased aorta, next to the heart, we started work at the upper end, near the branches to the brain and arms.

It was now nine thirty in the morning, and the operation was well under way. We had the aortic arch wide open. We had the brain's blood vessels entirely disconnected. We had a lot of work to do at the top of the aorta—and still more work to do at the bottom end, where we had to attach the coronary arteries to the new graft. Those are the small branches that provide blood flow to the heart's own tissues, and attaching them is a delicate and intricate task. And when all of that work was done, we would then need to rewarm the patient, a gradual process that would take at least an hour. Finally, we would need to stitch up the incisions and staple the breastbone back together. All in all, we were looking at another four to five hours of intense work.

At that moment, everything changed in our operating room. Everything changed in the United States, and in the world. Everything changed because this was the morning of Tuesday, September 11, 2001.

———

In any operating room, there are two nurses. The one called the scrub nurse stands at the table with the surgeons. She is responsible for preparing the instruments and sutures and providing them to the surgical team so they never have to look up and away from the operative field. The second nurse is called the circulator. She does not wear a surgical gown and she has not scrubbed up to the state of sterilization. That is because her job is to circulate around the OR, handling equipment, supplies, and machinery and coordinating with the blood bank and the ICU. At times during a procedure, she may go outside the room to retrieve supplies from the stockroom or the dumbwaiter that brings up equipment from the sterilization facility several floors below. Both positions, scrub nurse and circulator, are posts of great responsibility.

Our circulator that morning was Ms. Patricia LaFond. Patty is a fiercely independent, demanding professional, totally focused on comforting her patient and ensuring a safe, secure outcome. She is of that breed of dedicated, highly experienced professionals who can easily intimidate the students, residents, and even VIPs who visit OR 15 on any particular day. And I had never seen her anything but unflappable—until that day.

She came back to the operating room after a short trip to the dumbwaiter, and when she spoke, everybody looked her way. For one thing, it was not like her to interrupt an operation when the patient was in deep hypothermic arrest, when every second counted and no distractions were allowed. But the news she brought was well out of the ordinary.

"They are bombing Columbia and NYU Medical Centers. We have been alerted to expect casualties to be transferred to Yale for care, that is, if we are not the next medical center to be bombed."

My assistant was our chief resident, Dr. George Tolis, Jr. He and I were working feverishly to connect the head vessels to the main graft. We didn't know what to make of Patty's statement. But we knew that we had to maintain our focus on the patient and the work.

From then on, each time Patty's work took her out of the room, she came back with other tidbits of information. Some were accurate; many ultimately proved not. That is how it goes in a developing emergency. Patty said she had had a moment to glimpse some distressing video on the TV in the lounge adjacent to the operating room. There was something about the World Trade Center. There was something about airplanes. Iraq was attacking us, it was said. The United States was mounting an insurmountable air attack. Nuclear weapons might be used. University hospitals were being attacked along the East Coast. Schools were being let out, so that children could be with their parents. Companies were being shut, so that employees could seek the shelter of their homes.

The snippets of information that we were receiving were only partially based in fact. They were largely inaccurate and distorted. But we were isolated in OR 15, with no other source of information besides the rumors and innuendos that Patty LaFond could snatch from her brief moments in the outside world as she came and went, doing her job.

Dr. Tolis and I were also doing our jobs, working diligently against the DHCA clock, not permitting ourselves to be distracted from the exacting aortic reconstruction upon which we were engaged. All the while, we fully expected to have the lights go out, to hear emergency alarms and calls to evacuate and, we feared, explosions. For myself, I wasn't feeling that I was trapped in the operating room with my patient. I would do my best to bring him through no matter what was going on. As long as I had light and instruments and colleagues, I would never abandon my patient. I had never in my life left the table while a patient was on bypass, not even for a bathroom break. I am sure that George Tolis felt exactly the same way

My only concern was my children and my wife. My son, Andrew, was in the eighth grade at the junior high in our neighboring town, and my daughter, Christina, was a senior in high school. I wanted desperately to know that they were all right. I wished I could speak to my wife, Peggy, who is always calm and collected and knows exactly what to do in even the most trying situations. But given the circumstances, there was no chance of getting any kind of word to them or from them. In more than twenty years of marriage, my wife had never once called me in the operating room. I don't think she would even have known how to do so. In the back of my mind, after my wife and children, my thoughts turned to my "baby" sister, who worked for one of the big investment firms in Manhattan. Was she okay?

I was sure Dr. Tolis was having similar thoughts; I knew he had a brother in New York. Yet he worked beside me and never said a word. He would never abandon a patient in need; he would never fail in his duty. He had inherited the surgeon's sense of values and dedication from his distinguished father, Dr. George Tolis, Sr., a renowned cardiac surgeon in his own right (and himself familiar with OR 15).

But there was one uncomfortable emotion I had to deal with. Others had said in advance that Mr. Oliva's operation was futile, that the risk was too high, that he could never survive a reparative operation. The aneurysm was too large and too extensive. The heart muscle was too weak to tolerate such extensive surgery. That had been the kind of talk going around the hospital regarding my patient; and in truth, nothing that had so far happened, as we proceeded with the actual operation, had emerged to contradict those predictions. Though we were all doing our best for him, I recognized that there was every likelihood that this would be Mr. Oliva's last day on earth.

So the question was going through my mind: With some kind of terrible emergency going on in the world outside, why was I doing a nearly futile procedure? I had hours and hours of surgery ahead, I did not know if Peggy and the children were all right, and I could not reach them to give them a father's words of reassurance. And for what? Because I was performing a procedure that probably would not be survived, on a patient with an insurmountable constellation of serious cardiac issues. In a way, at least momentarily, I felt foolish and annoyed with myself.

Yet Dr. Tolis, the nurses, the anesthesiologists, the perfusionists operating the heart-lung machine, and I all persevered. We got the head arteries attached. This allowed us to begin circulating Mr. Oliva's blood through the heart-lung machine again—ending the period of suspended animation. He had been in the deep freeze for thirty-five minutes, well within the safety zone. We attached the coronary arteries, the right and the left, to the main graft. Then we hooked up the upper aortic graft to the lower aortic graft, restoring continuity of the arterial tree.

Now we started the process of rewarming the patient. Warming takes a long time—at least an hour, and more for larger patients like Mr. Oliva, who was heavy. We cannot warm up a patient who has been under suspended animation quickly—just by cranking up the thermostat on the heart-lung machine's heat exchanger. Human blood contains a great deal of albumin, a protein that is dissolved in the blood. The word "albumin" may sound familiar; you have probably heard that the white of an egg is composed of albumin. And thus you will know what happens to albumin when it is heated, as when an egg white is poured on a hot griddle: it yields scrambled eggs. Liquid albumin, when heated, turns into a solid. (This is technically called "denaturing" of the protein, changing its three-dimensional molecular structure.) So if we were to turn up the thermostat, we would cause the albumin in Mr. Oliva's blood to solidify, filling his bloodstream with the equivalent of scrambled eggs. This would block the arteries, resulting in stroke, heart attack, failure of all organs, and death.

So despite what was going on in the outside world, despite our fears and worries as fresh rumors and crumbs of information came into OR 15, we had to stand and wait. Waiting is not easy, especially for a cardiac surgical team. We tend to be doers, and doers make for poor waiters. Up until now, we had been working feverishly against the clock, cutting and suturing under the golden hour that deep hypothermic circulatory arrest allowed us, when every split second counted; now we had to stand, twiddling our thumbs, waiting for the gradual rewarming of Mr. Oliva's tissues.

I did not need an assistant while rewarming, so I sent Dr. Tolis out to call his brother in New York City. The nurse and I could handle most any contingency that might arise. He came back just a few minutes later and scrubbed back in. "My brother is okay," he said. "Dr. Elefteriades, you should go call your family. I can keep an eye on the heart. Don't worry; it will be okay." I had been toying with the idea of breaking briefly to call my wife. Fresh and disturbing rumors about what was going on in New York City and the world had kept coming into the operating room. I had never before realized just how isolated an open-heart OR can be, how completely insulated from the external world. My concern for my wife and children had been growing. Yet I had never—never in five thousand cases—left the operating table while a patient was on the heart-lung machine.

But I did so now. I "broke scrub," as we say, went to the phone in the locker room, and called home. Peggy was there. She was expecting Andrew and Christina on the bus. Word on the school district's telephone phone tree was that all students were being sent home. My wife and I spoke briefly about how to reassure the children, but she needed no input from me on that front; she knew instinctively how to handle emergencies. "I'll be home as soon as I can," I said, "as soon as our patient is safe."

Scrubbing up again before reentering the operating room, I was thinking to myself that I might be home very soon indeed. I fully expected the heart to fail when we attempted to come off bypass, given the very weak state of Mr. Oliva's heart muscle before the operation and the magnitude of what we had done to replace the aorta, its branches, and the aortic valve. All of that work had required more than three hours on the heart-lung machine.

After an hour and five minutes, Mr. Oliva was warm enough. We restarted the heart with a shock. On TV, that is portrayed as the critical juncture. In real life, the most critical point is when the burden of circulation—the load factor that comes with pumping blood to the whole body—is transferred from the heart-lung machine to the patient's own heart. That is the moment of truth.

Now that moment arrived. The anesthesiologist had started a heart-strengthening medication in advance, in preparation for coming off bypass. We decreased the speed of the pump; some of the load was thus transferred to the patient's heart. The heartbeat was adequate for a while. Then we began seeing signs of strain. My heart sank; I silently chided myself for taking on a case with an almost certain adverse outcome. But the private dialogue going on in my head reminded me that this pleasant, innocent man would have had no chance to survive if we had not taken him as a patient.

We started another heart-strengthening medication. The

heartbeat picked up again. We weaned a little more of the burden from the heart-lung machine. In a few moments we weaned further still, allowing the heart to adjust gradually to the task of circulating blood. A few more minutes passed in this way—gradual loading—and then we were off bypass fully. And successfully! Minute by minute, the heart grew stronger and stronger. The organ now began to recover from the strain of the operation and to benefit from having a brand-new, watertight, artificial aortic valve.

Mr. Oliva continued to stabilize. The echocardiogram showed already some tangible improvement in his heart's pumping strength, the ejection fraction discussed above.

We closed Mr. Oliva's chest successfully and transferred him to the ICU. I watched him closely for two hours, together with Dr. Tolis. Then finally, I drove home. On the way, I noticed a change in the on-road demeanor of the drivers around me. In a moment of national crisis, we Americans were banding together in an air of cooperation—petty differences set aside in view of the threat that had unexpectedly struck at us from beyond our borders.

———

I got home, and as was probably the same for you and your family, we planted ourselves in front of the TV and saw it all happen—incredulous, grieving, concerned for the future of a world population that could perpetrate the atrocities displayed vividly on our screen.

While my children, my wife, and I were watching, my sister

called from New York. She had been on her way to a meeting at the World Trade Center at eight o'clock in the morning, when suddenly her cell phone rang. One of the participants was unavailable, so the meeting was canceled and rescheduled. She turned her car around and headed back to Connecticut. But for that cancellation, she would have been in the World Trade Center at 8:30 a.m. on Tuesday, September 11, 2001.

Mr. Oliva made an uneventful recovery and was discharged into the care of his loving family five days later. He gave us all a hug along with his handshake and warmed us with his infectious smile. He had had no idea—how could he have?—of the individual drama that had played out in Operating Room 15 at Yale-New Haven Hospital while the horrific drama of 9/11 was playing out in New York City and the world.

I saw Mr. Oliva in a follow-up in my office about a month after his operation. He was doing exceptionally well. His color was good, and he felt healthy. His blood tests and x-rays were fine. The remaining diseased aorta was behaving itself. His liver was working properly, now that appropriate blood flow from the heart was restored. The new artificial heart valve was working well. The weakened, stretched heart was slowly improving in strength and configuration.

I sent a report to his superb referring heart specialist, Dr. Mark Grogan, of Derby, Connecticut, and in addition to the medical aspects, I commented: "I am just very, very pleased with

Mr. Oliva's recovery. It is nothing short of miraculous that he is alive and doing well. I told him that God was watching over him on that day, to have him survive and do well."

This case affected and moved me in many ways. First and foremost, I was deeply affected by Mr. Oliva's bravery. He understood that he faced stiff odds, yet he went forward with courage. Further, I was amazed that he survived the operation, with so many strikes against him. And I was absolutely incredulous that he made a good subsequent recovery.

The timing of the operation—right smack in the middle of the 9/11 attacks—was also very telling to me. An exceptional drama was playing out in New York City, in a field in Pennsylvania, and in our nation's capital—a drama that has changed our worldview forever. But in the very same span of time, during those fateful minutes, a smaller drama was playing out in Yale's OR 15—smaller, but no less a matter of absolute life or death. A human being was struggling for his life against incredible odds. For Mr. Oliva, and for the people who loved him, it was as dire a situation as it was for those who were caught up in the horrors of 9/11.

Mr. Oliva ended up being a survivor, through his own strength, and through the help he received from many dedicated individuals. I must ask you to remember, reader, that as terrible as the true events of 9/11 were, the terrifying rumors and scraps of information that came to my team while we worked on Mr. Oliva in OR 15 were even worse. We were first told that hospitals were being bombed, and that ours might be next. Yet no one, not the nurses, not the anesthesiologists, not the perfusionists, and not Dr. Tolis nor I hesitated to stay at our posts during the critical episode of DHCA suspended animation—when Mr. Oliva was clinically dead, but capable of being restored to life.

Every one of us stayed put and did our jobs while the worst disaster on American soil in our lifetimes was occurring just eighty-five miles down I-95. Each member of the team put Mr. Oliva and his needs ahead of their own and their families'. To me, this sacrifice was a tremendous manifestation of the human spirit, of dedication to the job of healing, and of truly caring for one's fellow human beings. I will never forget what my team and I were up to when the planes struck the towers.

Nothing stands still in the world of medicine, especially in cardiac care. About nine months after his urgent heart operation, Mr. Oliva developed a skin infection on his leg. It was treated, but eventually it led to a fungal infection of the bloodstream, where it took hold on his new graft and his new valve. Artificial hardware in the body is always susceptible to any infection that spreads through the bloodstream. When it latches onto hardware like what we had put into Mr. Oliva, so extensive and so intimately attached to the heart and aorta, there is usually no cure. We saw Mr. Oliva about the hardware infection, but surgically, there was nothing we could offer. We and his local doctors treated him with prolonged courses of antibiotics, first by vein and then by mouth. We knew that this treatment could at best only suppress and not cure the problem. Mr. Oliva battled on as best he could, but six years after 9/11, he succumbed to the fungal infection and was lost.

Mr. Oliva did not deserve to have the overwhelming heart disease with which he originally presented to us. Once he made it through the operation successfully, he did not deserve to develop a fungal skin infection and to have this go on to infect his cardiac hardware. He was a good man, leading a good, upstanding life.

Philosophers, and this heart surgeon, who studied philosophy before choosing a career in medicine, have for millennia pondered this question of why God lets bad things happen to good people.

Responses take two general paths. Some point out that without hardship and death, mankind would be bored and would not appreciate life. Others point out that we may be seeing just part of the picture, "through a glass darkly," and that innocents who leave us may be going to a much better place. This mystery will probably never be solved. But perhaps someday mankind may learn the truth.

Film Crew in the Room—Reflections on "Performing Live" on Camera

The patient in this vignette was operated on with the technique of deep hypothermic circulatory arrest (DHCA), which is a fancy technical term for "real-life suspended animation." This was pioneered by the fearless, creative Dr. Meshalkin, in Siberia—where there was no dearth of resources for inducing cold. In the early 1960s, he operated on babies with holes in the heart under real-life suspended animation induced by body immersion in cold fluid and snow.

At Yale University, we have amassed over the last fifteen years perhaps the largest contemporary experience with DHCA, with excellent clinical results. The public has been fascinated that these patients are clinically dead, with no pulse, blood pressure, blood flow, EKG (heart waves), or EEG (brain waves) for the duration of the DHCA. Multiple magazine articles and TV shows have been filmed at Yale regarding these techniques.

The science writer Colleen Shaddux spent days with us in the operating room for her article in the BBC magazine *Focus*; she entitled the article "Dead for an Hour: Patients That Are Dying to Be Saved." A corresponding article appeared in the U.S. version of the BBC magazine, called *Knowledge*.

We had three different film crews come to Yale—to the operating room, no less—to film one-hour specials for their TV shows. Imagine the added pressure for the team of knowing that these high-risk procedures were being filmed by TV crews. Above and beyond the obvious concerns, one never knows just how a newspaper, magazine, or TV show will use their footage. Fortunately for us, all the cases went well and the three programs produced excellent educational and entertaining segments.

The BBC came first. They were so bright, so animated, and

so involved that they became, for three days, members of our team. We worked together, ate together, and bonded powerfully. The show appeared worldwide on the acclaimed BBC TV series *Horizons*. I felt lonely when this remarkable, brilliant, inquisitive team left our university.

The Italians from RAI, one of the private Italian stations, were quieter and stayed more briefly. I have always been fascinated by Mr. Berlusconi, the controversial prime minister at that time. I had just read a biography of him, highly critical like so much in the U.S. press. Any questions I asked our film crew about their prime minister were answered with brief, noncommittal responses. Unusual, I thought, for Italians not to talk. I guess Mr. Berlusconi was, at the end of the chain of responsibility, their boss. One was probably fearful to speak openly.

Little did I know that, just a few weeks before these paragraphs are being written, I would actually meet Mr. Berlusconi! He attended our faculty dinner after a cardiac symposium in Milan. I found him engaging, warm, and fascinating. He even sang a long song for us (he started his career as a shipboard entertainer). It is easy to see how he won the hearts and votes of Italians, over and over again, despite his widely touted judicial and personal indiscretions.

The third crew came from the Science Channel, filming for the acclaimed program *Through the Wormhole with Morgan Freeman*. We found out that Mr. Freeman has been a science buff his whole life and, in addition to narrating the shows, is involved with their development and content. What a pleasure it was to have this crew, as well, join us for several days.

Like all their programs, the segment they filmed with us was presented in an entertaining yet informative manner. Unexpectedly, I received an invitation to a "cast party," if you will, at Mr. Freeman's residence. I was on a plane early in the morning, attended the party in Malibu in the evening, and was back to New Haven by the following morning via the red-eye from LAX. What a thrill it was to meet Mr. Freeman. He is much taller than he appears on film—and very polite and personable as well.

of physics at Yale. I had been told that he was very distinguished.

Chapter

4 Robert Ludlum

TWO HUNDRED MILLION BOOKS, AND COUNTING

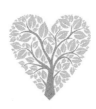 This is a story that needs to be told in three parts.

Part 1: *Hello, Sir. I Am Honored to Meet You*

One of the fascinating moments in the life of a surgeon is the first encounter—the moment you walk into a room and see the patient on whose heart you will soon be operating.

I have certainly had my share of unusual first encounters. I will mention a few before I go on to the patient who is the subject of this chapter.

In one case that I remember well, my patient was a professor of physics at Yale. I had been told that he was very distinguished, that he had just missed getting the Nobel Prize, and that the Physics Society had just honored him with a *Festschrift*—this is a German word for a book written to celebrate someone's career (usually with a corresponding celebration party). He needed an aortic valve replacement. After I introduced myself and we shook hands, we made some small talk. I usually ask about the patient's current or former profession (heart disease is more common after retirement age), and a bit about their families. That not only breaks the ice but also gives me a sense of the person I'm dealing with.

In answer to the first question, the patient told me that he was a theoretical physicist. Yes, I said, I had been told that. We spent a few moments working out whether or not, earlier in his career, he had taught me physics in my freshman year at Yale. We decided that it was possible.

Next, I asked him, "What is your particular specialty in physics?"

His response took me aback, especially considering that most patients do not want to antagonize the individual who is about to stop, cut, and rearrange their heart. In fact, as in psychiatry, there is usually an immediate transference reaction: patients want to think, and quickly come around to thinking, that their surgeon is the best in the region.

But my eminent physicist was the maverick in the herd. "I could tell you what I do," he said, "but it would be a waste of your time and mine. You couldn't possibly understand."

Ouch! I had studied a lot of physics and done quite well with it, as a matter of fact. But the distinguished professor obviously thought I was not bright enough to understand anything about his work. That point of view runs counter to my perception of scientific and medical research. I believe that if you cannot explain your research project to the average person in one or two sentences, you are not clear on what you are trying to achieve.

In the end, the professor did fine with his operation, and we became friendly. I got to meet many of his colleagues—indeed, quite a few of them came under my knife. I always took the opportunity to ask these accomplished theoretical physicists many of the fundamental questions about the universe with which I had been struggling for years. How does the Big Bang explain anything? How did the materials for the Big Bang get there in the first place? How did the energy get there? Do you believe in God?

What I've come to understand is that the answers to these deep, fundamental questions are as far beyond the grasp of the human mind as the workings of a computer are beyond the intellectual capacity of a squirrel. Even these brilliant theoreticians were not really any closer to the answers than you or I or the man on the street.

Another patient was also familiar to me from my early academic years. He needed a coronary artery bypass graft, the "cabbage" procedure described in Chapter 2. Years before, he had been Yale's dean of students, which meant that he had been in charge of my postgraduate career plans and was the person who actually signed my medical school diploma.

Of course, there was nothing unusual about my operating on a former teacher. What was unusual here was that, as we sat and discussed his case, I had a precise recollection of my long-ago interview with this dean—now to be my patient—when I was finishing medical school and applying for residency. His words are as clear to me right now as they were when he spoke them to me several decades ago.

"John," he said, peering over his reading glasses and leaning over the desk toward me for extra emphasis, "you have an excellent mind. I cannot allow you to waste it by going into surgery."

At that time, especially at schools like Yale, there was a strong prejudice in favor of internal medicine—thought of as a highly "cognitive" specialty—and against surgery, which was dismissed as the realm of simpleminded "cowboys" who wanted to just cut and never have to think. It has been a long struggle over the ensuing decades, but I believe the worldwide surgical community has proven its intellectual worth and finally overcome this prejudice.

And now, here I was, eleven years after graduation, being asked to perform the delicate task of a coronary bypass operation on the very dean of students who had told me bluntly that I should not be permitted to pursue becoming a surgeon. I was sorely tempted to remind the dean of his words, but respectful as always, I held my tongue.

The dean was actually an exceptional and caring individual.

He did fine with his operation, and lived on well into old age, taken care of perfectly by his bypass operation without a single further chest pain, heart attack, catheterization, or cardiac hospitalization for the rest of his natural life. It really is a miraculous procedure, the CABG, even if it was developed and perfected by "cowboys."

But now we come to the patient who is the subject of this chapter. Again, I can remember walking into his room as if it were yesterday.

Put yourself in my place. You walk into a room and there before you sits one of the world's greatest contemporary authors, a man many have called a flat-out genius. What do you say to someone who has sold two hundred million books worldwide—some of them to you, and you devoured them avidly—and who is still going strong?

What do you say when you walk in to meet and operate on Robert Ludlum?

Like millions of other airline passengers, I had hardly ever taken a plane flight without one of Mr. Ludlum's books in my hand. His plots were so intricate and engaging that I often wrote notes on the inside covers, just to keep the names of the characters straight, and to keep track of the main and secondary plotlines.

My good friend and colleague, Dr. Jeffrey Bender, had called to ask me to see Mr. Ludlum, to consider a coronary bypass operation. Jeff is medicine's answer to Derek Jeter: he can do anything as well as, if not better than, anybody else. First, he has the special acumen and clinical curiosity that make him a superb clinician. But, second, he is also an accomplished researcher, having built a distinguished investigative career studying blood vessels—and specifically the innermost layer, called the endothelium. His abilities have won him an endowed professorship at Yale. Jeff is a friend of the Ludlum family, and when Mr. Ludlum developed a cardiac illness, he became the patient's *de facto* cardiologist.

Dr. Bender told me that, at sixty-three years of age, Robert Ludlum was a mildly obese white male who smoked and drank heavily, and who was presenting with unstable angina. He had been admitted to the CCU (the Coronary Care Unit, where patients with serious, acute cardiac conditions are placed) with unstable angina. "Unstable" means just what the word says; "angina" means pain in the chest of cardiac origin. The chemical tests confirmed a heart attack. He also underwent a catheterization—in which dye is placed through a catheter, or tube, into the coronary arteries—and it showed severe narrowing of all three main vessels that feed the heart.

The arteries that would be targeted for a coronary bypass operation were not in good condition: they showed diffuse arterial disease throughout, with no good soft spots for the "touch down" of bypass grafts. There had been prior damage to the heart muscle, depriving the left ventricle—the organ's main pumping chamber—of about 20 percent of its normal strength. The pO2 (oxygen level in the blood) was only 69; it should have been 100.

This reflected the severity of the damage done to the lungs by years of nonstop smoking. One of the carotid arteries (the ones supplying the brain) also had a 90 percent blockage, which meant that surgery would carry a significant risk of stroke, causing brain damage. That was a possibility that I found especially worrisome. I dreaded the thought of operating on Mr. Ludlum and doing harm to that extraordinary brain that had beguiled and entertained people all over the world.

When I walked into the hospital room with "Robert Ludlum" on the door, I cannot say that I was intimidated, but I was deeply respectful. I expected an intelligent, complex man, and I was not disappointed. The adjectives "exceptionally smart," "absolutely intuitive," "worldly-wise," "proud but not arrogant," and "dignified" all come to mind. I found Mr. Ludlum not aloof, yet not warm either. Perhaps the spy business tends to purge whatever warmth is originally present. Also, I must use the adjective "brave." The more intelligent and knowledgeable the patient, the more vividly he conceives the potential dangers, and the more he worries about heart surgery. Mr. Ludlum knew that cardiac surgery carried risks. But his heart needed more blood flow; or else further heart attacks would follow. He bravely accepted that an operation was necessary and that we needed to proceed.

The operation was a triple bypass—much like in the procedure performed on Dave Brubeck in Chapter 2. We used the heart-lung machine and stopped the heart. We performed three bypasses, one with the mammary artery from inside the chest and two with veins from the legs. We warmed the heart back up and then shocked it back into a rhythm.

After an operation, the first concern of the cardiac surgeon is the heart itself: Will it pump well enough to support life? In the case of Mr. Ludlum, much to my relief, the heart began to pump, and pump strongly. Mr. Ludlum was transferred from the OR to the Intensive Care Unit in good condition.

The second concern is for the brain: Will this patient awaken well, able to move arms and legs, to follow commands—that is, with no stroke? In this patient's case, the gravity of this issue was compounded by two major factors: First, he had a narrowed carotid artery, which raised the risk of some adverse brain event. Second, Mr. Ludlum's splendid career, his special gift, and his extraordinary contributions to the world were all based on the intricate, complex outpourings of his exceptional intellect.

A patient usually takes a few hours to awaken after anesthesia for cardiac surgery. I spent the hours after sending Mr. Ludlum to the ICU trying to occupy myself in my office: seeing new patients, answering correspondence. Later in the afternoon, I could wait no longer. I went to the ICU and found that his blood pressure and pulse were fine. Oxygen level and blood count were fine.

I went to the bedside and whispered in the patient's ear, "Mr. Ludlum. Can you hear me?" Imagine my relief when he opened his eyes, I saw recognition in his gaze, and he nodded in the affirmative.

Thank God, I thought, *he has woken up properly*. He experienced some transient confusion over the next few days that we attributed to alcohol withdrawal, but then that cleared entirely. His breathing was a bit labored, as was to be expected from his underlying lung damage; but by the day after the CABG, he was able to breathe well on his own and was separated successfully from the ventilator that had been breathing for him. This had been yet another special concern in Mr. Ludlum's case, because of the lifelong heavy smoking and the low preoperative pO2.

The surgeon never breathes totally comfortably himself until a high-profile patient like Mr. Ludlum goes home. Mr. Ludlum spent several nights in a regular recovery ward, and on each of those nights I hoped the phone would not ring with any of the myriad of problems or issues that can arise. On the eighth post-operative day, he was ready for discharge, in excellent condition. Understandably, I breathed a sigh of relief.

I didn't see him get collected, but the nurse who took him to the hospital's circular drive told me that, true to form, Mr. Ludlum's driver had his limo waiting for him, and in it were three items: a carton of cigarettes, a bottle of Johnny Walker, and his latest girlfriend. Mr. Ludlum was living up to his legend.

For me, I felt a special privilege at being afforded an opportunity to get to know—and care for—one of the great authors and storytellers. I was exposed firsthand to a first-rate intellect. It was my privilege to care for his heart and, with my team, to restore him to heart health. I was truly humbled by this experience.

As well, this case gave me experience with yet another high-profile, world-leading individual, which contributed to my comfort with other VIPs who were to come my way in the future.

Mr. Ludlum showed his kindness, his gift with words, and even, as you will see, his dry sense of humor in thanking Dr. Bender, our Yale team, and me. His next novel was Apocalypse Watch, *and this is the dedication:*

A Note from the Author

I've rarely written a dedication more than two or three lines. This current one is different; the reason is self-evident.

To the brilliant cardiologist Dr. Jeffrey Bender, MD, and the superb cardiothoracic surgeon Dr. John Elefteriades, as well as the surgical crew and all those in the CTICU of Yale-New Haven Hospital, whose skill and concern passeth all understanding. (Although it could be argued that I was a glorious patient—although not very convincingly.)

Now let's lighten up; there's always something funny even in the worst of times. During a perfectly normal sponge bath a day or so after surgery, a kindly nurse turned me over and with great dignity, as well as a glint in her eye, said: "not to worry, Mr. L., I'll still respect you in the morning." Amen. And to all once again, my deep thanks. I'm ready to run in a marathon.

So I was honored to have had a spot in Mr. Ludlum's life. I thought that was the end of that story.

Not so.

I keep on the wall of my office the letter Mr. Ludlum sent me after his recovery. I treasure this along with other memorabilia from both the famous and the ordinary (but the ordinary are never ordinary at all).

During the last few days before he left the hospital, Mr. Ludlum was well enough to have conversations with me. Sometimes, when I visit a patient to talk, I sit on the corner of the bed. I believe it can be comforting and reassuring for them, breaking down the distance that can develop between doctor and patient. But not with Mr. Ludlum. I simply felt too great a respect for him to be so familiar. I sat on the chair by his bed and we talked.

I was keenly interested in the creative process. "How do you do it?" I asked him. His replies stayed vividly in my mind and were, as we will see, to serve me well some years later.

"It's easy," he said. "The central idea, the kernel, if you will, is the framework. That framework is like a coatrack, on the rungs of which you simply hang characters and plot." Easy for Robert Ludlum, I thought; not so for mortals.

"And how do you get that kernel idea?"

"That I don't know," replied Mr. Ludlum. "That just comes into your head. And you have to know your subject. I am a spy, and I know the spy business. That is why I write spy novels."

A few moments afterward, he said, "Doctor, you know heart surgery. You should write a novel about heart surgery. You know medicine inside and out. Other writers need to research their subjects with the experts. You will be a giant step ahead. I know you can do it."

No wonder he was such a great novelist. His author's intuition had sniffed out the motive behind my questions. I could see that he read people well. How could it be otherwise, given the vividness of his characters?

Like so many doctors, I had always felt the attraction of fiction writing. I had always loved language and languages, probably because I was raised bilingual. My parents had come from Greece as very young adults. I was born in Philadelphia. My mother spoke perfect English with a lovely British-Greek accent, and had a superb vocabulary. She was also fluent in French, having distinguished herself in high school in Greece after the Second World War.

Yet my parents chose to speak to me only in Greek until I was old enough to start school. My mother was confident that I would quickly learn English in kindergarten, and she was right. I walked into my first school not knowing a word of English, but within a week or so, I had amassed the small vocabulary of the five-year-old. From there on, I grew up knowing two ways of expressing my thoughts—the Greek and the English—and I am sure that that ability contributed immensely to my fascination with language. I have always loved grammar, vocabulary, and syntax.

In high school, I studied French and Latin, enthralled and

mesmerized by their grammatical structure—although I must admit that my dedication to *la belle langue* had something to do with the fact that my teacher, Mrs. Borick, was not only a warm, nurturing woman, but also an absolutely voluptuous beauty. The rumor that we teenaged boys passed around was that she had given up the glamour of being an exotic dancer to become our French teacher. It never occurred to us that such was an unlikely career path in a quiet suburb of Philadelphia.

I continued to study French at Yale. I just loved the language and the classics—Molière, Racine, Corneille. I was encouraged to continue the study of French literature in graduate school, and there were even hints that there might be a place for me on the teaching staff at Yale after I finished. Until the very end of my undergraduate years, I strongly considered going for my PhD in French literature. What a difference that would have made in my life. But my father, the practical mechanic, discouraged that option, with the argument that acquiring expertise in classical French dramatists and novelists might not be the best preparation for a career in the real world.

So I became a doctor. But in-depth study of French grammar contributed to my command of English grammar. And I continued to love to write. I pride myself on the clarity of my medical and scientific writings. But writing for the general public, that's a different story. I started with two nonfiction books aimed at the general public: the first entitled *Your Heart: An Owner's Guide* and the second *The Woman's Heart: An Owner's Guide.* I was proud of those, especially the first, from which the second derived. Those two books represented the first dips of my toe in literary waters, in terms of writing for a general readership.

About ten years after I met and cared for Mr. Ludlum, with his words of advice still reverberating in my ears, I started to work on a fiction book. I had had that "kernel" core idea in my mind well before the day I sat in Mr. Ludlum's room to get his advice. Now, finally, I was working from that kernel, my coatrack, and adding characters and plot, as Mr. Ludlum had recommended. "Easy" he had called it, once you have the kernel idea; just add characters and plot.

Not so for me. Not easy at all. I stayed true to Mr. Ludlum's advice to "know your topic," so I made the protagonist a heart surgeon—what profession could I possibly know better? Furthermore, I built the story around a core that was also in my "sweet spot" of knowledge and experience: an ethical issue in cardiac transplantation. The heart surgeon who is the book's protagonist is a talented but substantially flawed character; you may draw your own conclusions from that.

Knowing exactly the core ethical issue with which I wanted to challenge my readers, I went ahead with characters and plot. I would sit in stolen moments and write as the words came to me. Saturday mornings were good; I could come back from my morning rounds and write for an hour or two before the family was up. I had only a novice's grasp of where to go with the characters and the plot; I just saw what happened at the keyboard.

My real job—heart surgery—is conducted in a world of harsh

reality. The patients I see are more than a little sick, and often their needs are desperate and their options limited. Fiction offered me a stark and enjoyable contrast: I could make anything and everything happen the way I wanted. I did not even need to overstress the reader's considerable capacity for suspension of disbelief.

Thanks to Mr. Ludlum, I began to lead a veritable "double life." I felt as if I had slipped into someone else's skin. By day, I was the heart surgeon I had always been. On weekends and stolen days, I was a fiction author. The experience took me to new and exciting places, with radio and TV interviews and magazine articles and newspaper write-ups. Suddenly, I was at the London Book Fair and at the New York Book Expo, with my name hanging from the ceiling and a line of readers, albeit an inconstant and small queue by comparison to those waiting to have their books autographed by the better-known authors. I felt honored, unduly, when someone wanted to read my book. I spoke to all of them about themselves and their interests.

I am happy (and very surprised) to report that the book, *Transplant*, did not receive a single negative review. It was used in an ethics course at the Medical School, and it even won a "Top Five" award for first fiction work. Go figure!

The second novel, again centering on an ethical dilemma in medicine, is being written concurrently with the nonfiction book that you are reading now. It takes place on the island of Santorini, thought by many to represent the lost continent of Atlantis, and concerns not transplantation, but rather, genetics.

I am confident that none of this "double life" would have occurred without the influence of Mr. Ludlum. It was his concepts of the "kernel" and the "coatrack" that got me through the process, not to mention the sheer inspiration that emanated from knowing him.

Part 2: *Pre-Death Obituary*

I had operated on Mr. Ludlum in 1993. It was now 2000. I was thrilled that he had done well. By this stage in my career, I was lecturing widely around the world, and it seemed that each time I turned around, there was another Ludlum bestseller on the shelves at the airport bookstore. I could only imagine how many more millions of books had been sold beyond the two million that Mr. Ludlum had achieved when I first met him. And by now there were the blockbuster movies—and a series of them, about the tormented secret agent Jason Bourne, played by no less a box-office draw than Matt Damon.

It was now eight years after his bypass operation. My phone rang.

Dr. Everett Alsbrook, who had been taking excellent care of Mr. Ludlum in Florida, along with Dr. Marc Mootz, had called Dr. Jeff Bender again about their patient. Mr. Ludlum had had no further difficulties with heart attacks or with his coronary arteries. That was to be expected, because the bypass operation is a tremendous procedure, honed to perfection over the years by medical science. Mr. Ludlum's CABG was taking great care of the blood-flow needs of his heart.

But other problems had developed. Mr. Ludlum had kept on smoking cigarettes: he admitted to more than two packs a day, and we should keep in mind that the admitted level of smoking usually underestimates the factual level. Mr. Ludlum was now having difficulty breathing after any exertion. He had been unable to do any exercise whatsoever.

Dr. Bender saw the patient in his office at Yale. As he put it in his report to the Florida physicians, "Mr. Ludlum has [developed] three advanced conditions, all potentially very serious. One is bilateral carotid artery disease, a second is severe chronic [pulmonary] obstructive disease, and the third is critical aortic stenosis." The term "bilateral carotid artery disease" meant that the arteriosclerotic blockages in the carotid arteries that provide blood flow to the brain had now worsened and come to affect both sides. It was an ominous sign. The term "severe chronic pulmonary obstructive disease" signified that the lungs had been permanently damaged by the many years of cigarette smoking; lung capacity was measured at about 40 percent of normal. Home oxygen therapy was being considered. The term "critical aortic stenosis" indicated that the aortic valve, the main outflow valve of the heart, had become blocked, essentially "choking" the heart.

Dr. Bender concluded that another cardiac surgery to replace the aortic valve needed to be considered, although, as he put it, "I am most concerned about the risk of surgery given his carotid disease and his severe obstructive pulmonary disease." Mr. Ludlum steadfastly refused any surgical intervention at this juncture—probably a logical posture given the exceptionally high risks. Second cardiac operations are always more dangerous than the first, even without the other risk factors mentioned by Dr. Bender, because of so-called "adhesions." That is, once a body cavity has been operated on, the tissues lose their normal anatomic borders; they all stick together in one conjoined mass; such is the reaction of body tissues after being exposed and manipulated. Risk is especially high when, as in Mr. Ludlum's case, the first operation has been a CABG, as the delicate bypass grafts themselves are highly vulnerable during reentry into the chest and surgical dissection of the various structures.

Dr. Bender even enlisted the support of the distinguished Dr. Kenneth Kearns, the patient's nephew and a leading gynecologist, in trying to convince Mr. Ludlum to have surgery. But Mr. Ludlum was resolute in his refusal.

Mr. Ludlum limped along, with the aid of home oxygen therapy, and with his physical activity greatly restricted. He gained weight from his immobility. Then, on March 29, 2000, he was admitted to his Florida hospital with heart and respiratory failure. There were now no other options, and the patient was transferred to Yale by air ambulance for reconsideration of ultrahigh-risk surgical intervention.

A cardiac catheterization was done. I held my breath. The surgeon "owns" for life the grafts he has created, and any problems would reflect on me. As I noted above, the target arteries in Mr. Ludlum's heart had been suboptimal due to the extensive and diffuse nature of the disease. Amazingly, the catheterization showed that all the bypasses were open and pumping beautifully—pristine. However, the aortic valve, as expected, was found to be critically narrowed. There was no alternative but surgery.

My colleague Dr. Richard Gusberg, a vascular surgery specialist, operated first, to clean out the right carotid artery. This procedure is called carotid endarterectomy. The carotid artery needs to be clamped while the endarterectomy is performed, and that always entails a risk of stroke. Dr. Gusberg was on tenterhooks, as I had been nearly ten years earlier, until Mr. Ludlum awoke. But the patient came to fully, his superior brain completely intact. However, due to local traction on one of the nerves next to the carotid artery, he was having trouble swallowing, and the excess secretions accumulating in his throat and dripping into his lungs further challenged his breathing. All of us thought that this should improve over time. We gave him a few days to recover.

Then we scheduled my turn at the operating table. I do high-risk cases every day, often exceptionally high-risk cases. Mr. Ludlum's case fell into the category of extreme risk; worse, many of the risk factors were beyond our control: the lung disease, the carotid blockages (the endarterectomy does not make all the disease go away), and now the swallowing difficulty that was jeopardizing his airway. I took a deep breath when the case was officially scheduled. My biggest fear was the definite risk that we might lose Mr. Ludlum on my watch.

I contacted Yale's public relations department and discussed the situation with them. I pre-wrote a death report so that they would have it on hand. I thought it was best to be prepared for the media attention—negative attention—that was likely to fall upon us; I did not want any reflection on Yale or on myself to ignore the extreme underlying risk of this situation. I wanted, essentially, to be prepared with a pre-death obituary, although I had never done this before in my career. This is what I wrote for the PR group to have ready for immediate dissemination:

Yale–New Haven Hospital, April 7, 2000—The distinguished author Mr. Robert Ludlum expired today during treatment at Yale New-Haven Hospital for end-stage cardiopulmonary disease. Mr. Ludlum had undergone life-saving coronary artery bypass surgery at our institution nearly ten years ago. His pulmonary disease and a new problem of aortic stenosis became acutely life-threatening, and he was air-lifted again to Yale, where he underwent urgent and extremely high risk reoperative cardiac surgery. His disease was overwhelming and he did not survive. Yale is proud to have participated for years in the care of this remarkable individual and to have prolonged his life as long as possible.

The pre-mortem obituary written and ready, we went forward with the actual operation itself. The operation was difficult. We preserved the pristine bypass grafts. We exposed the aorta safely. We replaced the valve with a mechanical valve. The patient survived. He awoke properly. Most amazing, he was able to breathe adequately on his own. The positive outcome outshone even my best possible expectations.

When he was well enough, Mr. Ludlum called for his airplane, and he was transferred again to the care of Dr. Alsbrook in Florida to complete his recovery. Miraculously, we did not need to use the preprepared press release.

We got early reports from Florida that, under Dr. Alsbrook's attention and with his insight and wisdom, Mr. Ludlum was recovering satisfactorily. I was greatly relieved. Mr. Ludlum was once again delivered safely from my watch.

I heard nothing further, but in such circumstances, no news really is good news.

Weeks and months passed. Then, on March 12, 2001, I returned to my hotel room in Liège, Belgium, after lecturing during the afternoon. I turned on the TV. Mr. Ludlum's face appeared on the screen, with a brief report that he had died in Florida of natural causes. I felt a deep sense of sadness for the great man's passing and a strong conviction that the world had lost one of its most remarkable intellects. I was relieved that the team at Yale had shepherded Mr. Ludlum safely through so many cardiac, vascular, and pulmonary issues. I felt that Yale had served Mr. Ludlum very well, given his natural limitations and addictions.

My life would be forever enriched by my having known and cared for Robert Ludlum. It was, for me, a true brush with greatness. I got to experience firsthand Mr. Ludlum's razor-sharp intellect, cutting humor, world-weary familiarity with the ways of humankind, and love of storytelling. Were it not for my meeting Mr. Ludlum and having him encourage me to write for the general public—and specifically to write fiction—I would never have had the experience of becoming a novelist, albeit as a rank amateur next to his greatness.

As well, this case served to harden me to the extra burdens that come from caring for the very rich and very famous. I have learned, in such circumstances, to call up my inner "ice man"—to forget the identity of the body on my operating table, and to concentrate on the anatomical and clinical and pathological aspects of the one square foot that is my whole world when I am fixing a heart.

Knowing Mr. Ludlum enriched my life in many, many ways. But that was not the end of the story.

Part 3: "The Ludlum Identity"

Readers of Robert Ludlum will recognize the style of the above title—an article, followed by a proper noun, followed by a common noun—that Ludlum popularized, beginning with *The Scarlatti Inheritance. The Ludlum Identity* is indeed the title of a book, and it is very much a Ludlum book—but not because Ludlum wrote it. He is not the book's author; he is its subject. And fittingly, it concerns a mystery.

It began, for me, nearly ten years after Mr. Ludlum's passing. I thought of him often, and especially every time I entered an airport bookshop and emerged with another paperback with a three-word title and his name on the cover. Even after his death, I was pleased to see that he had left behind so many unrealized ideas for thrillers that others could complete for him.

The Risks of Reoperative Cardiac Surgery

The famous patient in this chapter comes to need a second cardiac operation. It is hard for the layman to imagine, but the risks of a second operation are much higher than a first.

First, just opening the breastbone on a second operation is hazardous. We open the sternum with an oscillating saw, but the previously operated heart can be adherent to the undersurface of the bone, making it vulnerable upon reentry. Injury to the heart upon reentry can be catastrophic.

Furthermore, any body cavity, be it thorax (sides of the chest), mediastinum (middle of the chest), or abdomen, reacts with what we call "adhesions" once it has undergone surgery. That is to say, the pristine glistening membranes that normally cover the heart and intestines become inflamed (irritated) and stick to each other. In the case of the heart, the pericardial membrane sticks to the heart surface. That can make for indistinguishable natural landmarks. The situation can resemble the old-school task of carving a boat out of a block of soap. The surgeon knows the normal anatomic distribution of vessels and chambers, and he uses that knowledge to facilitate carving the heart out of the adherent structures. Of course, *this is dangerous, as cardiac chambers and structures can be injured, sometimes seriously or irrevocably.*

Finally, the dangers are especially great when there are bypass grafts (either vein grafts or mammary artery grafts) surrounding the heart. You might think that the bypass grafts would be clearly apparent and thus safe, but such is far from the case. In fact, the grafts become enmeshed in the general adhesions in the pericardial cavity, and they can easily be injured. Such injury can be life-threatening—not only because the graft will bleed, but also because the segments of heart muscle supplied by that graft will be deprived of blood flow and lose contractile function.

All these dangers were vigorously in play when the famous author in this chapter came, in bad condition, for his second operation. That is part of the reason why we preemptively prepared a pre-mortem obituary statement.

Then, one day, when I was in my office, catching up on a stack of written correspondence that had accumulated on my desk, I found something at the bottom of the pile.

It was an invitation from Dr. Kearns to a November fifth signing event for his book, the full title of which is *The Ludlum Identity: The Man Behind Jason Bourne.* The formally printed card included an intriguing invitation to "join in a lively discussion related to the life and mysterious death of the famous novelist Robert Ludlum." The words "mysterious death" captured my attention immediately.

It was already November third when I happened to find the invitation and I read those words. There was no telling how long the invitation had sat, unnoticed, on my desk. Almost all my correspondence these days is by e-mail.

I was intrigued by the words "mysterious death of the famous novelist Robert Ludlum." I had always presumed—although I had never investigated—that Mr. Ludlum had died from his pulmonary disease and other chronic medical problems and addictions, and I had never given a thought to any other possibility. Now, I wanted to know, what could possibly have been "mysterious" about Ludlum's death?

I recognized right away the name of the distinguished Dr. Kearns, Mr. Ludlum's nephew, whom I had met during Mr. Ludlum's hospitalizations. He had served on the Yale faculty and then moved to Scottsdale, Arizona. Now, it appeared, he had written a book about his uncle's life and especially about his demise. The event was to be held in Simsbury, about an hour from New Haven. I e-mailed Dr. Kearns to see if, at this late date, I could still respond affirmatively to his invitation. Yes, of course, he said. He assured me that I would find the information he was presenting very interesting, and that his book contained substantial documentation that called into question the verdict that Mr. Ludlum's death had been "natural."

I told him I would order his book right away. And I did. I have had it on my shelves for several weeks, but at the time I am writing these words, I have not yet read it.

I wanted to complete this chapter based on my own documents and recollections—without influence from whatever additional information I might find in Dr. Kearns's book. I wanted my report to you to be uncontaminated and uninfluenced by any new facts or interpretations of those facts. While I was writing this chapter, I must admit that I reached for the book several times, but each time I mustered my surgeon's self-discipline and put it back on the shelf.

But now I have completed the story of how I met and came to know the great man and to participate so intimately in his cardiac surgical care. Now, at last, I will read his nephew's book. You the reader will not notice any passage of time, but the next line you read will have been written some considerable time after this one.

———

Well, let me say it right off that *The Ludlum Identity* is a terrific read. Dr. Kearns provides an insight into Mr. Ludlum that only someone who was close to him as a member of his family and as his de facto personal physician could deliver. He gives a sense of Robert Ludlum, the man in full: the entrepreneur, the ladies' man, the dreamer, the risk-taker, the multitalented author/spy/ thespian, the entertainer, the raconteur, the confabulator, the world traveler, the keen observer—a much more multidimensional rendering than I had ever appreciated. He conveys how deeply and truly Mr. Ludlum loved his wife, Mary, "more than anything else in the world." She was his "anchor." I felt Mr. Ludlum's grief and despair at her passing, and I could understand his desperate longing for a companion to fill the huge void left by her death.

When I heard, while I was in Belgium, that Mr. Ludlum had died, I presumed that the liquor, the cigarettes, and the multiple physical afflictions had simply caught up with him. But Dr.

Kearns's book recounts his "discovery of extremely disturbing information relating to Robert Ludlum's life in the months preceding his death" and regarding the exact mechanism of his death. My original impression, and that of the public, may have fallen far short of the mark.

How far short? My reading of *The Ludlum Identity* raised a strong suspicion that criminal forces may have brought on Mr. Ludlum's death. The machinations and complexities of his passing take on a surreally sinister complexity that would not be out of place in a Ludlum novel.

I recommend Dr. Kearns's book very, very strongly. I was fascinated by the new perspectives he opened on Robert Ludlum's life and by his exposition of the apparently criminal forces that were at play in his death. Among the fascinating insights (and I quote directly in some instances):

- Robert Ludlum's true birth identity remains a mystery.
- He was abandoned after birth and adopted.
- His military record, or lack thereof, generates suspicion.
- Serious questions surround Mr. Ludlum's will, which involved last-minute alterations and multiple suitors for his fortune and empire that was worth, even at a conservative estimate, hundreds of millions of dollars.
- Mr. Ludlum is not buried where the media say he is.
- There was no funeral, either public or private.
- Mr. Ludlum's remains were cremated immediately after his death, precluding any forensic analysis of the cause of death.

- Above all, Dr. Kearns maintains that Mr. Ludlum's demise was ultimately "Death by Unnatural Causes."

Both as a doctor and as a writer, I was impressed by the way Dr. Kearns lays it all out, with the key documents reproduced in their entirety. His is a fascinating book. Any Ludlum enthusiast—and we are many—owes it to himself to read *The Ludlum Identity*.

For me, the revelations in Dr. Kearns's book had a personal impact. I had presumed that my best efforts had ultimately failed to combat the cardiac and other ailments that plagued Mr. Ludlum. Naturally, that engendered a degree of disappointment; I would have liked him to have gone on living—and especially, writing. Now I have to take into account the possibility that the reality may have been very different. Dr. Kearns's book would seem to indicate that, were it not for the maneuverings of nefarious forces, Mr. Ludlum might well still be alive today.

Chapter

5

Still Life

"THERE IS A YOUNG WOMAN ON THE PHONE . . ."

Written with Shireen Dunwoody and the
assistance of Anne Merrit

Bless your uneasiness as a sign that there is still life in you.

—DAG HAMMARSKJÖLD

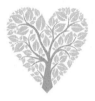 I was sitting at my desk, having just finished a coronary bypass operation. I was starting to look over the items in my physical "in box"—requests for references for graduates of our training program, hospital forms, administrative memoranda.

Lorena buzzed me. "I am sorry to disturb you, but there is a young woman on the phone. She says she had surgery here twenty years ago, and she doesn't know what was done." Lorena had astutely put the young woman on hold, while she retrieved the office file. "You are going to want to see this file," she said, with excitement and a twist of mischief in her voice. "It is Isalia Alvarez on the phone."

The name didn't click—how could it after ten thousand

cases—but it took just a momentary glance at the file to bring back the most powerful of memories. I was overwhelmed with incredulity that Isalia could possibly be alive and well enough to be calling on the phone. Could it really be true? How could I possibly explain the past to her?

I pushed the flashing button on my phone and said, "Hello, Isalia. Do you know anything at all about what happened?" What I didn't say was that I could not believe that she was alive, let alone well enough to call.

A Terrible Accident

On an unusually cold January day in 1987, Isalia and her family were in a devastating car accident on Interstate 95 in Guilford, Connecticut. Isalia was just four years old at the time. Her father, mother, and two brothers, Mark, twelve, and Caesar, eight, were also in the car. The story was reported the following day by *The New York Times*. I have deleted certain parts of the article so that I can describe some aspects of the event in my own words.

From The New York Times, January 21, 1987:
DARING RESCUE IN FRIGID RIVER SAVES 8-YEAR-OLD
by Dennis Hevesi

A former New Haven police officer and a New York City fire-fighter were credited yesterday with a daring rescue in which they pulled an 8-year-old boy from a submerged van that was being dragged into the frigid currents of a Connecticut river.

The boy's mother died of heart failure at St. Raphael's Hospital after the accident. [His] father, brother and sister [were] considered "basically dead" when brought to Yale-New Haven Hospital.

A spokesman for the Connecticut State Police, Sgt. Daniel Lewis, said the accident took place at 3:42 P.M. Monday, in the westbound lanes of Interstate 95, near the town line between Madison and Guilford, Conn.

Van Becomes Submerged

"The highway was very icy," Sergeant Lewis said, "and the van vaulted over the cables and landed in the East River," which flows south into the Long Island Sound.

"The entire van was submerged about 25 feet from the shore," he said. "There was about 18 inches of water running over the top of the van."

The former police officer, 39-year-old Robert Ramadei of Northford, Conn., said he was driving home when he saw the yellow van, driven by Caesar A. Alvarez, 40, of 132 Guy Lombardo Avenue, Freeport, L.I., "spin out of control and crash through the cable." It was Mr. Alvarez's son, Caesar D. Alvarez, that Mr. Ramadei and the firefighter, Barry Meade, 37, of Port Washington, L.I., are credited with saving.

Mr. Ramadei said he ran down the embankment but by the time he got near the van, the current was taking it further into the river. "I could hear the people screaming and I knew there were children in there," he said.

Grabbing an Ankle

Mr. Ramadei swam out to the van. "The vehicle was totally submerged," he said. "I dove down to the passenger door and I could not open it. The terrifying thing was that I could see the people and they were in a total panic situation. I swam to the driver's door. I was unsuccessful in opening that door.

"I then swam to the top of the van, which was 18 inches under water. There was one of these crank-open vents. I smashed that with my hand. I had to submerge my right arm and head to reach in and feel around. The interior was full of debris. Thank God, I came up with Caesar's ankle. And I pulled him through by his ankle."

By then, Mr. Meade, a scuba diver with the City Fire Department's Rescue Co. 1 in Manhattan, had swum to the van with ropes from his car. "I reached into the van and tried to find anyone else I could reach," Mr. Meade said, "but the hole wasn't big enough.

"The child wasn't breathing," he said. "Bob gave him some back compressions, and the child cried. He mumbled, 'Mommy, Daddy.'"

With the rope, Mr. Meade said he tied Mr. Ramadei and the boy together. "Bob swam the child to shore, with people on the shore pulling them in," he said. "I only wish we could have gotten the rest of the family out."

Sergeant Lewis said emergency crews managed to secure the

van with cables. "They had people in cold-water survival suits," he said. "By breaking out one of the windows, they reached inside and pulled out three more people"—Carmen Alvarez, 32; her son, Mark, 12; and daughter, Isalia, 4. Later, a state trooper found the father.

Sergeant Lewis said Mr. Ramadei and Mr. Meade "really took a chance."

"It only takes a few minutes in waters of that temperature when you're not equipped with cold-water gear to lose control of your own muscles," he said. "They certainly are heroes."

Hypothermic Resuscitation

On that fateful day in 1987, we had just finished operating in the Cardiac Corridor, Rooms 15, 16, and 17 at Yale-New Haven Hospital. In that era, ordinary operations, even a coronary artery bypass procedure, took nearly all day. The heart-lung machine had not been perfected, control of medications to thin and then thicken the blood were still suboptimal, and the techniques for hooking blood vessels to each other were not as well sorted out as they are now. So operations took a while, especially at a teaching hospital, where young physicians were learning by doing, under faculty tutelage. Anyway, all the rooms were just free at four o'clock in the afternoon. All the surgeons who had been operating that day were still in the vicinity of the operating rooms.

We had recently resuscitated a patient who had been frozen in

Connecticut's frigid winter, so the stage was set for the call that was about to come in. Dr. Grahame Hammond, one of our senior surgeons at the time, and one of my own cardinal mentors, got a call from the emergency room. "There is a frozen family being brought in from I-95. Do you want to try to resuscitate them?" The emergency response team at the scene on the highway had heard about our recent success with a frozen person and wanted to know if we would try to save this family from their desperate circumstances. Dr. Hammond had the typical cardiac surgeon's brash bravado from that era. His response was, "Bring them right up."

So Dr. Hammond rounded up those of us who had been operating that day and called us back to the operating rooms. I was the junior man on the team at that time, just a few years out of my training. I reported to my Room 15, and the father was wheeled in. Dead. My colleagues Dr. Hammond and Dr. George Letsou manned Rooms 16 and 17. Isalia and Mark were brought into those rooms. Dead. None of the three patients on our tables had a pulse, a heartbeat, an EKG, or any level of consciousness. They were about 73°F, having been quickly cooled by the icy waters.

It had been a family of five. The mother had been taken to St. Raphael's Hospital, a neighboring facility two miles from our own; she had died there. The middle son, Caesar, eight years old, had been successfully revived at the scene; he had been the first one grabbed by the ankle by Mr. Ramadei and brought out through the upper hatch. The others were not extricated until quite a bit later, when help and heavy winch equipment had arrived. Isalia, four, and Mark, twelve, were on our operating tables now. Their father, also named Caesar, was on my table.

All three of our emergency patients had been blue, unconscious, and without pulse or blood pressure at the scene. Cold water immersion times had been thirty to sixty minutes, depending on the order of extraction. None of the three were breathing spontaneously. A breathing tube had been placed for each one, and artificial respiration and CPR begun.

Beyond those initial measures, we did not know exactly what to do. We were three separate surgical teams in three different rooms and we were not in contact with each other.

As it turns out, all three surgical teams independently took the same tack. We splashed a bit of antiseptic on the skin and "crashed" into each patient's chest, dividing the breastbone down the middle with a saber saw. We quickly put in a retractor to separate the bone edges, and we placed large tubes to connect to the heart-lung machine—one to carry the patient's spent blood to the heart-lung machine, and another to carry the fresh, pressurized, oxygenated blood back from the heart-lung machine to nourish the patient's brain, heart, and other organs. And we did this as quickly as possible—for each patient had been without blood flow for many long minutes since the heart arrested in the cold waters of the Connecticut River.

We had precious little experience with resuscitation from hypothermic cardiac arrest. No one in the world had substantial experience. We were on uncertain ground—applying extraordinary measures in a likely futile endeavor.

As we circulated blood with the heart-lung machine, we "turned up the heat"—that is to say, we slowly dialed up progressively warmer temperatures on the heat exchanger that is an integral part of the heart-lung machine apparatus. The heart cannot beat unless it is at least 89°F. But we had to rewarm the body slowly, as too rapid rewarming makes the blood literally curdle—a devastating phenomenon. (See Chapter 3 for more on rewarming from deep hypothermia.)

So with the patients attached to the heart-lung machine, warming slowly, the immediate pressure was off the surgical team. The frenetic action to open the chest and hook up to the machine had been completed. Now we needed to be patient, to see what, if any, results would be had.

When we compared notes later with the teams in the other operating rooms, we discovered that much the same procedure had been followed in each case, with the exception that in my room, rewarming took considerably longer, because the father of the family was by far the largest patient of the three.

We recorded starting temperatures of 71° to 79°F upon initiation of warming.

In all three rooms, as the body temperature rose above 90°, we witnessed the very same amazing phenomenon. Each heart stopped its frenetic fibrillation and took a tentative beat. After a long pause, another beat was seen. As seconds grew into minutes, a steady succession of beats ensued. *The "dead" hearts had reestablished their rhythm.*

We still knew nothing about the strength of the heart or

about the patients' brain function and other organs. We allowed each heart to warm further, to bask in the warm, oxygen-rich blood from the heart-lung machine.

When we reached full warmth (after one to three hours, depending on the patient's size), at about 98°F, it was time for the acid test. Could these revived hearts possibly sustain the circulation? Could they fulfill the body's need for blood flow without the artificial support of the powerful heart-lung machine?

Little by little, in tandem in each room, we gently transferred the burden of circulating the blood from the heart-lung machine to the patient's own heart—essentially "weaning" from the machine, like weaning from a mother's breast. Much to our surprise, with patience and care and support, each heart—the father's, Isalia's, and Mark's—was able to meet the challenge. Each patient was successfully weaned from the heart-lung machine.

As our distinguished chief of staff of Yale-New Haven Hospital, Dr. John Fenn, put it later for *The New York Times*: "These people arrived basically dead. No pulse, no blood pressures, no respiration. Their temperatures were approximately 73 degrees. Medical teams managed to restore the heartbeats of Mr. Alvarez, Mark and Isalia."

All three patients were transferred to Intensive Care Units, Mr. Alvarez to the Cardiothoracic Intensive Care Unit, and the two children to the Pediatric Intensive Care Unit (ICU).

We had no idea what to expect in terms of potential survival or neurologic function—no data or substantive experience from which to prognosticate. We only knew that because these patients had arrived dead, we and they, in the most ultimate terms, had nothing to lose.

Mr. Alvarez survived for several days. Being by far the largest physically of the three, he had cooled the least effectively. That is to say, his internal organs did not benefit as much from the preserving power of the cold temperature of the Connecticut River as had the physically much smaller children. Mr. Alvarez showed all the effects of cardiac arrest and oxygen deprivation. He never regained consciousness. While his heart beat satisfactorily, his lungs filled with water, reflecting damage to the cell membranes from his cardiac arrest and the resulting inadequate blood flow. When the body cells do not receive nourishing blood flow and oxygen for a time, the cells are injured, and their membranes, their protective outer coatings, leak precious fluids out of the cells and into the surrounding tissues. Mr. Alvarez deteriorated progressively and died within seventy-two hours after his drowning.

The situation was different in the Pediatric ICU. The children, much smaller physically than their parents, had cooled their brains and internal organs much more effectively in the frigid January river currents. Each child showed some signs of brain function. Their cell membranes appeared okay. Their lungs did not flood with fluid. Their liver, kidneys, and other internal organs revived fully and worked well.

Over time, each of the two children regained some—although nowhere near full—brain function. Each did become alert enough to be weaned from the ventilator (the breathing machine) and breathe normally and spontaneously. Each child had evidence of neurologic damage. This included incomplete recovery of cognitive skills and some abnormalities of sensation and movement of the extremities.

Nonetheless, we were pleased and astounded at the children's mere survival. Both Isalia and Mark were stable enough that they were able to be transferred to a rehabilitation facility. I held out hope for their continued survival. I expected that there might be some slight additional neurologic recovery—after all, children are incredibly resilient—but I did not expect much. We received some limited, but encouraging, news from rehab in the early weeks, but I suspected this was all wishful thinking, because of the circumstances. I doubted I would ever hear much additional encouraging news.

In fact, I heard nothing, nothing at all. Until twenty years later, when *Isalia was on the phone*.

A Call Twenty Years Later

You can imagine my surprise, my shock. Isalia was alive! She was twenty-four years old. She was well enough to talk on the phone, and *she sounded normal!* She knew she had had some kind of operation twenty years ago, and she was calling me to find out what it had been. She was so young at the time that the scar had healed and was barely noticeable, but it was there; she knew something surgical had been done. I explained the amazing story in broad strokes, sensitive not to shock Isalia any more than necessary while remaining truthful to the events of twenty years earlier. How do you tell a twenty-four-year-old that she was clinically dead at the age of four? How do you recount the sad family tale without inducing horror, panic, and sadness?

Isalia remained composed and unemotional. She and her brothers had been raised by family members, she told me, and they had overheard a word or two about what I described. And, she told me, Caesar was alive and serving his country in Iraq, and Mark was also alive and doing well. I was flabbergasted. I never expected neurological recovery. Absent neurologic recovery, long-term survival was extremely unlikely. I was beside myself with amazement and gratitude for the survival and functional recovery of these children from a horrendous accident that had occurred in the dead of the Connecticut winter fully twenty years earlier.

This was a truly amazing medical and human story.

I kept my wits about me enough to ask Isalia, at the end of our conversation, if I could tell her family's story. Her affect was rather flat. She had no objection.

Mark has no memory of the accident. He said that when he fell asleep in the car, his parents were there, and when he awoke in the hospital, woozy and somewhat disoriented, he learned his parents were gone. He feels he is physically healthier than most other young people, yet he still experiences the sadness of losing his parents and having to uproot his life at such a young age. He did undergo some physical therapy for injuries to his left hand and, because he was left-handed, had to learn to write with his right hand for a short period. His left hand is fine now. Although he knows his brother, Caesar, was conscious throughout the accident, he said they have never spoken about it. Mark is now happily married and living in Austria with his wife and his dog.

As reported in *The New York Times* article, Caesar was rescued at the scene by Robert Ramadei and Barry Meade. He remained in touch with both rescue heroes for several years after the accident. Caesar is currently a major in the U.S. Army in the 304th Military Intelligence Battalion, which is considered the home of military intelligence leader training. In addition, the 304th Military Intelligence Battalion writes tactical intelligence and electronic warfare doctrine, and conducts advanced training programs to prepare Army leaders who are proficient in advanced intelligence skills.

The story of this family is a vivid demonstration of the protective powers of cold. Cold preserves the function of the brain and other organs by decreasing the metabolic needs of the body tissues (the amount of blood flow and oxygen required for cellular activities). Under normal circumstances, when the brain is starved of oxygen, cells start to die *within four minutes*. After five minutes, there is a good chance of permanent brain damage. In a way, Isalia and Mark were in a state of real-life "suspended animation." The case of the Alvarez family informed the medical profession that resuscitation was possible in such circumstances and has led to multiple other stories of salvage of the otherwise "dead."

Real-Life Clinical Application of Suspended Animation in Cardiac Surgery (See also Chapter 3)

Real-life suspended animation is applied daily at our hospital and selected others throughout the world. This technique was originally developed in Siberia, where ice and cold are never far away, for use in babies with "a hole in the heart." In the fifties and early sixties, before the heart-lung machine became available, daring Russian surgeons put babies into an ice bath until their hearts stopped. The cold temperature protected the child's internal organs while the surgeons put the baby on an operating table, quickly opened the chest, and placed a stitch or two to close the hole in the heart. They then closed the incision quickly and rewarmed the baby in a hot water bath. As the baby warmed, the heart restarted, and the patient awakened to a normal life, forever cured of the "hole" in the heart and its otherwise debilitating or life-threatening consequences.

Today, we use hypothermia routinely for complex surgery on the aortic arch, the part of the aorta that gives off branches to the arms and the brain. We produce real-life suspended animation at a temperature of 18°C (or 64°F). During this time, we shut off the heart-lung machine—and the patient is without EKG (electrocardiogram, or heart wave trace), EEG (electroencephalogram, or brain wave trace), pulse, blood pressure, or blood flow. In other words, there are absolutely no signs of life. We can invariably safely sustain this state for nearly forty-five minutes, and usually sustain it safely for sixty minutes.

Cold is remarkably protective of biological tissues. The metabolic rate falls as temperature decreases—meaning that very little blood flow is required to keep an organ alive at low temperatures. The drop in metabolic rate is not linear, but rather, exponential; that means that the metabolic rate falls much more rapidly than the temperature decreases. In other words, hypothermia is very, very protective. The patients undergoing aortic surgery via this technique awaken normally, with fully restored cognitive function—memories, abilities, instincts, etc. We often find the patients reading their favorite novels or magazines by evening of the same day.

Because of our specialized program in aortic surgery at the Aortic Institute at Yale-New Haven, we have accumulated one of the largest experiences in the world with the hypothermic suspended animation technique—called technically "deep hypothermic circulatory arrest."

The fact that patients do so well, with all their cognitive functions, memories, skills, instincts, and talents intact, leads me to surmise that storage of information in the brain must be "hard-wired" in some way, so that the relevant "connections" are preserved even without energy (blood flow).

Multiple media programs have reported on our real-life suspended animation program, including the BBC magazine *Knowledge* as well as the BBC television series *Horizons*, Italian RAI *Voyager*, and the Science Channel's *Through the Wormhole with Morgan Freeman*. This topic of cheating death via hypothermia—"You are not dead until you are warm and dead"—is fascinating to the general public.

Questions and Answers with Dr. Elefteriades
(Interviewer: Shireen Dunwoody)

Q. *Do you think there is a particular reason why the case of this family is so significant to you out of all the cases of hypothermia resuscitation you have performed?*

A. Well, of course, it is unique, as it involved an entire family. We truly didn't expect any of them to survive. You can imagine my shock when I received the call from Isalia. Following our resuscitation efforts, the children were both sent to rehabilitation. Although we had done our best and the children survived, at that time my expectations of the outcome were fairly low, as they had been submerged for a long period. I wasn't at all sure if they would survive after hospital discharge, much less to be able to function well enough to carry on a conversation. They were both lost to follow-up. So, you can imagine my immense surprise when I learned that both Mark and Isalia had survived and were functioning adults.

I have to tell you that it wasn't until I began writing this chapter and discussing certain aspects of the accident that I understood how it may relate to an incident in my own past. As a sophomore in college I had worked extensive overtime at the U.S. Post Office during the summer to purchase a 1967 Corvette Stingray 327 that I was able to restore and rebuild. I was so proud of that car. My classmate at Yale had a 428 Cobra Mustang. Needless to say, we had quite a bit of fun with those vehicles.

At that time, Yale did not yet accept women. On alternate weekends, Yalies would visit the women's colleges and the women would visit Yale. On this particular Friday in October, we were headed to Vassar College in Poughkeepsie, New York, which at that time was an all-female institution. I was in the Corvette and my friend was ahead of me driving his Mustang. Believe it or not, on this particular day we were actually behaving ourselves, as the roads were icy and wet. However, as we approached a small two-lane bridge over a river, I could see that my friend was running into trouble. The back of his Mustang started to fishtail and he was losing control of the car. Because I was behind him, I had time to brake. When I hit the brake, my Corvette immediately started to fishtail badly out of control. In an instant, I was spinning in complete circles along the icy road and had lost all control of the vehicle.

In what must have been just seconds, I saw my entire life, the whole thing, flash before my eyes. It was just as others had described it. In that moment, I knew I was going to die.

When the car finally stopped, I was inches from the bridge rail and perfectly parallel parked. I have no idea how that happened. When I stepped out of the car, I was so frightened my legs buckled beneath me. I didn't die, but in that moment when the car was spinning *I knew I was going to die.* In other words, I suddenly had an awareness of my own death. Until that time, death wasn't real to me. I was only nineteen so that's understandable, but I was truly changed after that day. I was aware of my own mortality. I had cheated death. My car didn't go into the water, but the story could have been so different.

I think this may be why the story of this family has haunted me. It so closely resembled this incident from my own past that could have ended in a completely different way. It could have ended so differently for the Alvarez family as well. In a split second, one decision made or not made, one action taken or not taken, and the fate of so many lives can be altered.

Q. *It must be very strange as a surgeon to have a patient on your operating table who is clinically, well, dead.*

A. Very much so. The last thing a surgeon wants to have happen is to have a patient die. The moment patients are placed on the operating table, the surgeon feels responsible for their lives and, in a worst-case scenario, for their death. I think this is true for every surgeon. Imagine, then, how unnerving it is to have a patient arrive clinically dead. There is no category for that. In every such case I ask myself if I should risk the heartache and potential moral and legal implications for what is usually only a glimmer of hope for survival.

Q. *How do you decide which patients to resuscitate?*

A. What I now understand is that death is on a continuum. There is a saying, that you are not dead until you are warm and dead. (In other words, if you are cold and dead, you may still be revivable, thanks to the protective effects of cold.) For a patient to be a candidate for resuscitation, there must be some sign, an occasional or intermittent heartbeat, a slight movement, that indicates they may survive. Also, it helps if the surroundings have been ice cold. Further, it is encouraging if the duration of cold exposure is known in some manner. After the initial case with Isalia and her family, Yale became known for providing hope in what would have been hopeless hypothermia cases. In the freezing Connecticut winters, I have been awakened many nights with calls for these types of patients. We have not always been successful. Unfortunately, some cases don't end well.

Q. *What are the key differences between deep hypothermic cardiac arrest (DHCA) and accidental hypothermia cases?*

A. The accidental cases are, by definition, completely unplanned and the circumstances of cold exposure, in terms of duration, location, and associated trauma, have a profound effect on outcome. We employ planned, surgical DHCA under very controlled conditions for a limited duration. Our team has experience with thousands of cases.

Q. *How did the care of this family affect you?*

A. It affected me in many, many ways.

My colleagues and I became involved firsthand in a terribly tragic event. As I have noted in other chapters in this book, I often grapple with the age-old question of why God permits tragic events to happen to human beings. My profession has led me to witness and become involved with these situations in an up-close-and-personal way. The mystery of why such terrible things happen occupies my mind. I doubt that human intellect will ever sort this out.

I also recognize the astounding bravery of the New Haven police officer Ramadei and New York City firefighter Meade, who are the real heroes in this case. How could anyone even venture into those frigid currents? How could the police officer break the roof vent with his fist? What an extraordinary degree of caring for one's fellow man these two men demonstrated! They did not hesitate to jump into a freezing river—with no protective equipment, putting their own lives in extreme jeopardy—in order to try to save people they did not know, a family trapped in their van under water.

To this day, I am moved, almost to tears, contemplating this extraordinary altruism. I am awed by the actions of these two heroes, which ultimately permitted the survival of three children, so that they could grow up and become fully functioning adults. Perhaps therein lies an answer to the question of why God lets bad things happen: to offer human beings an opportunity to show how good we can be.

This case demonstrates for me the crucial importance that a split-second decision can have for a patient's outcome. Dr. Hammond, when he received the call from the emergency room, could very well have said, "We can't help this family. They are dead and gone." No one could have reasonably questioned such a response.

Yet he did not make that call. In a split second, he said, "Bring them right up."

Were it not for that instantaneous judgment call, two lives—Isalia's and Mark's—would have ceased at that moment. Instead, they have gone on for another twenty years.

Probably, above all else, this case demonstrates the extreme courage and resilience that these three children must have mustered to survive after a tragedy of this magnitude. God gave them the strength to meet the great challenge of losing their parents at such a delicate age—and the challenge of coming as close as humanly possible to losing their own lives. Yet they overcame.

I hope that, as you have read this chapter, you have been moved to share in my fascination with the reality that death can be cheated by hypothermia. This topic has tremendous philosophical, medical, and religious connotations.

Chapter 6

Wendell Minor

TRIUMPH AFTER ADVERSITY

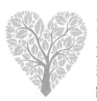 It is summer in 1964. A young man lies in a hospital bed in a major Chicago medical center. He is the child of Norwegian and German parents, both of whom were raised in an Illinois farming heritage. He has just turned twenty. He was operated on six days previously. He is recovering. He feels a bit dizzy and a little euphoric. The "high" comes from his relief that he has survived a surgical procedure that was new, dangerous, and far out on the fringe of established practice.

Although his head is spinning, the young man can tell that one of the cardiac residents, on routine rounds, is standing by his bed. What the young man cannot see is the worry that seizes the resident as he detects something he doesn't like. The resident sees pallor in the young man's face and does not like the thready feel of the patient's pulse. A glance at the collection chamber on the floor by the bed shows that a liter of blood has drained out of the man since morning rounds, and a steady stream threatens to overflow the capacity of the container.

The cardiac resident makes a decision. He calls to the nurse, "Get blood." He shouts to the nurse's aid, "Call a Code Blue." The resident feels perspiration collecting on his forehead. His armpits are getting moist. But he knows his job. He is rational and composed as he moves to the end of the bed and pushes it with all his strength toward the operating room. He knows that the young man's life lies in the balance. Every second will count.

The young patient has seen considerable adversity during his short life. Since childhood, he has had a heart murmur. Accordingly, he was prohibited from participating in sports. In the Midwest, in that era, to be prohibited from playing baseball or football was tantamount to ostracism—so much of school life and status in the teen hierarchy revolved around sports. Adding to the adversity, the young man had had trouble with his schoolwork since grade school. He had been put in remedial classes for reading and math. He had felt "dumb" for his entire life up to this very point. Had we known fifty years ago what science knows now about information processing in the human brain, we would have recognized soon after he started school that this young fellow had suffered from dyslexia. Today, we would identify the condition and correct its impact before any heavy emotional damage was incurred.

But this young man had drawn strength from his adversity. Since as far back as he could remember, he had been able to do one special thing: *he could draw.* He knew he had talent, and he worked hard to nurture and enhance his natural ability. He was mature enough to understand that he was not the only young man in the world who had artistic talent. If he wanted to distinguish himself—to be the "go-to guy" for all things artistic—he had to work hard to hone his skills. This he did. He became precisely the go-to guy. At school, he became the one they turned to when they needed posters, banners, book covers, mascots, or illustrations for the school magazine, or sets for plays. For all of these, his classmates and teachers came to him. He was something of a phenomenon in his community.

"That Wendell Minor," people would say, "he sure can draw."

But in that Chicago hospital bed in 1964, Wendell Minor sure was bleeding. Six days before, he had undergone surgery to repair a coarctation of the aorta. This is a congenital narrowing of the aorta, the main artery of the body. This narrowing, usually located at the top of the chest, just beyond the artery to the left arm (called the left subclavian artery), prevents blood from flowing smoothly and freely to the lower body. As a consequence, the legs have little stamina, and running becomes nearly impossible. Also, the constriction puts a great strain on the heart, which has to pump against a blocked outflow artery. To complicate matters further, as a result of a physiologic link via the kidneys, coarctation causes premature hypertension, or high blood pressure throughout the body.

Six days before, surgeons had cut out ("resected") the narrowed portion of the aorta and replaced it with a Dacron tube about an inch in diameter and three inches in length. In that era, such a procedure was always an adventure and carried substantial risks.

Perhaps the greatest of those risks was bleeding, and that was what the cardiac resident concluded was happening right now to young Mr. Minor. The patient himself was feeling mellow, because he was on his way to unconsciousness, as blood leaked out of his aorta and his blood pressure fell. The blood was coming out through the two large, garden hose–sized tubes that are routinely left in the chest. These are left specifically to drain blood and fluid that is routinely shed during the recovery phase. Now, however, the tubes were filling at an alarming rate. The cardiac resident knew that the young man would lose consciousness soon and that cardiac arrest and death would quickly follow suit.

The bags of blood from the Blood Bank now arrived, and the resident and nurses started rapidly transfusing, hoping to match the bleeding cc-for-cc to prevent exsanguination ("bleeding out") and death. Right now those bags of blood were all that stood between Wendell Minor and death. As we will see later, those bags of blood were to have lingering effects, ultimately becoming a risk to his life—and to mine. But for now, Mr. Minor's bed was still being rushed down the hall to the operating room, even as the resident and nurses tried to keep him from bleeding to death. Ironically, the patient was originally scheduled to have his stitches removed the very next day. Instead, other events were unfolding.

In the operating room, the anesthesiologist was waiting, and the nurses were quickly preparing their table with the instruments and sutures that would be required for an operation called a "reexploration for bleeding."

The patient was placed with his left side up, the skin was quickly splashed with Betadine (an iodine-based antiseptic), and the resident started taking out the sutures placed in the incision six days before. He took out first the skin sutures, then those in the underlying fatty layer (subcutaneous tissues), then the sutures in the muscle layers, and finally, those holding the ribs together. Blood gushed out of the chest, over the sterile drapes, onto the floor, and onto and even into the resident's shoes. A full sweat now broke out on the young surgeon's brow. Residents in cardiothoracic surgery in that era were confident—the fighter pilots of the surgical world—but still, the resident found himself hoping that the attending surgeon would arrive soon.

As the resident cleared blood and clots from the chest cavity, he placed a retractor to separate the ribs. "Suction," he said to the scrub nurse. With the aspiration device, she sucked at the base of the wound and now the aorta came into view. There was a vigorous bleeding site where the Dacron graft had been sutured to the patient's own aorta.

Just then, the attending surgeon came barging through the

door, fastening his mask as he burst in. "What's going on? What happened? Talk to me," he shouted to the room. He was brought up to date as he took his place to the left of the patient.

The attending held finger pressure on the bleeding site while the resident loaded his stitch. One well-placed mattress-type suture fully controlled the bleeding. Stability was restored. The patient survived. The resident's rapid recognition of the bleeding event and his immediate, decisive response to this emergency situation had saved Wendell Minor's life.

So let's recap. By the age of twenty, the young patient had lived through a difficult childhood, being dyslexic and finding himself excluded from many activities because of his heart murmur; he had been subjected to a major surgical procedure for coarctation of the aorta, and then he had survived massive postoperative bleeding that took him to the brink of death. Adversity and a life lived on the fringes of normal adolescent culture had already given him a mature outlook on life. Now, at much too young an age, he had just survived a very close brush with mortality. That was the sort of near-death experience that can imbue the survivor with a permanent sense of overwhelming gratitude for the gift of living every day and every minute that had almost been snatched away.

Young Wendell Minor already possessed a precociously mature sense of appreciation for life. Unlike most young men of twenty years, he did not feel invincible. Not so for Wendell. He knew the value of each and every moment of life that he had been granted, and he wanted to savor every minute of time he had been allotted, as well as to make his mark on the world.

Before these life-threatening events unfolded, Wendell had just completed his first year in a nonaccredited, super-intensive three-year art program. During that first year, Wendall had experienced bouts of nearly passing out, severe headaches, nausea, and vomiting (all symptoms of his coarctation). After the aortic operation, complicated by bleeding, followed by a prolonged, difficult hospitalization, Wendell was told he could not possibly return to school. He needed to "rest" for a year before he could even consider any activity. Wendell, who now saw every moment as a precious gift, had no intention of wasting time by doing nothing. He would have no part of such a plan. He returned directly to art school—to the intense but unaccredited Ringling School of Art in Sarasota, Florida. He had a sense—he knew already—that art would be his route to personal fulfillment, to recognition, and to contribution to society. He was back in school immediately, savoring every moment and building up his "drawing muscles" substantially day by day.

In his senior year at Ringling, Wendell was recruited by Hallmark Cards, and before long, he was drawing professionally for Hallmark in Kansas City and then for the legendary book cover designer Paul Bacon in New York City. He worked at Paul's studio for a year and a half, until Paul decided to downsize his studio and go solo, at which point Wendell began to look for other job possibilities. This led him to Random House, where he had an interview with Robert Scudellari, the corporate art director. He did not get the job for which he interviewed, as the art director told Wendell he simply had too much talent and needed to work for himself, in order to realize his maximum potential.

To make a long story short, Mr. Minor, as I will call him from this point on, became one of the most highly regarded contemporary artists and illustrators in the country. I had been made somewhat aware of this by the time I met him in consultation. Later in this chapter, I will share additional information about his accomplishments that subsequently came to my attention. I should point out as well that Mr. Minor honed his didactic and oratorical skills in many years of teaching art at the collegiate level intertwined with his illustrative work.

Mr. Minor had risen to the apex of contemporary American art by the time that I met him and his lovely wife, Florence, a supremely talented woman in her own right. They had met at a dinner party that Wendell had not wanted to attend. They were instantly attracted, they bonded, they married, and they have been inseparable for thirty-seven years. Florence, a writer, former film editor, and speaker in her own career, plays an integral role in Wendell's work. She serves as his No. 1 critic, so closely linked to her husband and his work that he describes her as "the side of my brain that really works." Mr. Minor and Florence consider each of his books their "children" together.

Florence and Mr. Minor came to see me in my office in October 2005. He was sixty-one years old. He had been diagnosed with an aneurysm of the ascending aorta. It was large. Surgery had been recommended, and I concurred fully. Mr. Minor had been referred to me by Dr. Adam Brook, one of our former residents, and an author in his own right (*The Golden Gate Diet: How to Lose Weight and Maintain Your Health, A Scientific Method for Weight Loss*). Mr. Minor had illustrated and designed Dr. Brook's book cover. His official cardiologist was the distinguished Dr. James Cardon, in Hartford, Connecticut.

In addition to the aneurysm, Mr. Minor had been born with a congenitally abnormal aortic valve, which had produced his childhood murmur. Most of us have three leaflets in our aortic valves, resulting in a "Mercedes-Benz"-type appearance of the valve leaflets. (The three leaflets split the circle into three equal parts, with their borders mimicking the Mercedes emblem.) Mr. Minor had been born with only two leaflets in his aortic valve, resulting in a "fish mouth" appearance of his valve. This two-leaflet valve morphology, called a bicuspid aortic valve, is the most common anomaly of any kind affecting the human heart. It is seen in one in every fifty human beings (a really common anomaly by medical standards). If you are sitting in a crowded movie theater for a popular first-run movie, several people sitting in the audience around you have this lesion, although they do not know it. Bicuspid valve alone accounts for more morbidity and mortality than all other congenital heart lesions combined.

You may be surprised to learn by whom a bicuspid valve was first described. This lesion was first noted—and beautifully de-picted in a drawing—in the fifteenth century by none other than the unfathomable genius Leonardo da Vinci. So great were da Vinci's talents and accomplishments—in art, engineering, science, and anatomy—that myths have sprung up about him— even the notion that he was not an ordinary human—that he must have been an extraterrestrial. If he was human, so the myths go, so great were his talents and vision that he must have been augmented or instructed by visitors to our world. I prefer to think that he was an example of how high our species can rise, all on our own.

Now Mr. Minor's bicuspid valve had worn out prematurely, as such valves are prone to do. Anyone's aortic valve can wear out after millions of openings and closings, say by the age of eighty or eighty-five. But bicuspid valves wear out much sooner, a couple of decades sooner, in fact. So Mr. Minor, at age sixty-one, had an aortic valve that had become narrowed, its normally supple leaflets having been infiltrated by calcium, the building block of bones, rendering the leaflets rigid and immobile. Instead of having a normal opening of 4 square centimeters (about the size of a quarter), Mr. Minor's valve was reduced to 0.9 square centimeters (about the size of the eraser on the end of a pencil). This has the effect of "choking" the heart. The muscular pumping chamber of the heart, the left ventricle, tries valiantly to pump blood through the aortic valve, but the narrow valve impedes the flow of blood, severely straining the heart muscle. Imagine your biceps trying to curl a 50-pound dumbbell instead of a 10-pound dumbbell. Or imagine the fuel pump in your car trying to work with its main outflow valve blocked.

Patients with aortic stenosis, a blocked aortic valve, do poorly without surgical correction. In fact, once they develop symptoms, they tend to die at an alarming rate over the next few years. The symptoms classically include shortness of breath, chest pain, or passing out. Yet aside from some fatigue, Mr. Minor continued to feel well despite his aortic stenosis—probably a testament to his high general level of fitness.

In my notes from his visit, I described the patient thus: "Mr. Minor keeps himself extremely fit, through a vegetarian diet and yoga." I also described in my initial consultation letter the impact of his early brush with death: "Mr. Minor had a coarctation repair in 1964 when he was twenty years of age, by Dr. Beatty. He had a very difficult time, with a cardiac arrest post-operatively, a massive hemorrhage, and a reexploration for bleeding. This left a very vivid and unpleasant memory in the patient's mind. He feels that every year since that time has been 'extra life,' and he has savored it."

I heard his heart murmur easily, and graded it at V/VI—the second loudest category possible. The murmur could be heard "radiating" loudly into both carotid arteries in the neck.

I noted, "In view of his very difficult experience with this coarctation surgery as a youngster, Mr. Minor has understandably been reluctant to have further cardiac procedures. Also, he is a 'homeopathic' sort." Mr. Minor did not rush into a decision in favor of heart surgery.

I saw him again four months later. Now the aortic valve's open area had decreased even further, to the critical dimension of 0.7

square centimeters. This exacerbated the already considerable burden on the heart muscle.

Also, by this time, a CT scan had been done on Mr. Minor—and it revealed another problem: The aorta above the bicuspid valve was massively enlarged, at 7.3 centimeters (the normal range is up to 3.8 centimeters). Aneurysm in this location frequently accompanies bicuspid aortic valve.

So for many reasons—because of the large aneurysm and because the congenitally bicuspid aortic valve had now become blocked—Mr. Minor needed major open-heart surgery. I indicated, however, that, respecting his frightful experience with cardiac surgery early in his life, having made my recommendation for surgery, "I will not pressure him in any way."

By the way, coarctation (for which Wendell had been operated decades earlier), bicuspid aortic valve, and aneurysm of the ascending aorta often are seen together as a cluster of abnormalities affecting a single human heart—a sort of "Combo No. 1" of congenital heart lesions.

There was, however, a complicating feature. Those units of blood that Mr. Minor had received forty-two years earlier had left a lingering effect. In those days, blood tests for communicable diseases were rudimentary. From those units, which had saved Wendell's life when the postoperative bleeding occurred, Wendell had contracted hepatitis C.

Mr. Minor had always had a "holistic" approach to his health. He watched his weight and his diet. Whenever possible, he preferred a holistic approach to an interventional one. By mind over matter, he had managed to live many years with no ill effects from the hepatitis C. (See the sidebar on this disease.) I found that quite extraordinary, and in this man who possessed a very special, very powerful mind, I consider this a true manifestation of mind over matter. Mr. Minor's viral counts had never spiraled out of control. Dr. Myron Brand, the respected Yale gastroenterologist, evaluated Mr. Minor's liver, finding it remarkably well compensated despite no traditional treatments having ever been given.

Ultimately, Mr. Minor decided to go forward with surgery—a remarkably heroic and brave decision on his part.

But that raised another problem, on my part—an *ethical* problem, and a thorny one at that. You see, we usually treat hepatitis C before cardiac surgery with powerful medications. These medications, while not ideal—in fact, they are difficult and somewhat toxic—can drop the viral load to zero in many patients. Mr. Minor really wanted no part of this. He had kept the disease at bay on his own, without drugs. He was not interested in pursuing traditional medical therapy now, not even as a prelude to the recommended extensive cardiac surgery that he plainly needed.

So we had a problem. I was concerned that liver dysfunction could add to the already significant risks of aortic replacement. I told Mr. Minor that I had to think carefully about whether I could offer him a corrective operation for his aneurysm.

Now I will be candid with the reader. There was another layer of complexity—another concern running through my mind, and one that I shared frankly with Mr. Minor. The hep C put myself and my team at considerable risk during the surgical procedure. Hep C is highly contagious. Give the virus the slightest chance to invade a new host, and it will take it. Cardiac surgery offers the hep C pathogen a whole raft of opportunities for transmission from the patient to the doctors, nurses, and allied personnel.

After all, for 4½ hours, we would have our hands and arms fully immersed in Mr. Minor's chest. Sure, we wear gloves and gowns, but tears and leaks frequently occur in the OR—often many times during a single case. If we the medical staff have any break in the skin, even a hangnail, the viruses can enter our bodies and proliferate, thus transmitting to us the hep C. Also, as we saw in the emergency operation that Mr. Minor underwent at the beginning of this chapter, cardiac surgery can be a bloody business. Blood often spurts, splashes, or spills—and viruses can enter the bloodstream of the staff via contact with eyes, nose, mouth, or any cuts or scrapes. Blood and blood-containing irrigation fluid often spill from the edges of the surgical field. Over the years, I have lost countless pairs of socks from such spills, and shoes as well. I have also lost underwear in this way, when a spill soaked through my scrub pants. (Fortunately, my wife has been very understanding of my coming home, on these occasions, with no underwear or socks.)

Keep in mind as well that, unlike surgery on other parts of the body, in heart operations the patient's entire bloodstream is removed from the body and circulated through clear plastic tubes to the heart-lung machine. The potential exposure of the staff is much more extensive than in noncardiac operations. The machine has many connections and ports from which samples are taken, offering still more opportunities for the viruses to spread themselves to new hosts. And there are plenty of prospective hosts, since at least eight people are in the room, all subject to potential contamination and contraction of this virulent viral disease: one surgeon, one or two assistant surgeons, a scrub nurse, a circulating nurse, two anesthesiologists, and two perfusionists. Furthermore, some of these individuals may go on shifts during the operation, or to lunch or break, thus exposing even more dedicated personnel to potential intimate exposure to the virus.

Moreover, needle sticks abound during cardiac surgery. They can happen during the intense concentration on the operating field for especially intricate portions of the procedure. They also happen very frequently when big, strong needles are used to pass heavy wire sutures (about as thick as a paper clip) through the breastbone for closure. Any such needlestick is a first-class ticket for the eager viruses into the surgeon, nurse, perfusionist, or anesthesiologist—another victim for the powerful, smart, ugly viruses hell-bent on frenetically replicating themselves in a fresh, new human host.

Of course, hospital administrators will say that, since historical times, physicians have exposed themselves to the potential dangers of disease via treating their patients. From the safety of their offices, which are seldom splashed with infected blood, the administrators will say that such exposure risks are "part of the job." In fact, surgeons may be subject to sanctions if they refuse an infectious patient. But any heart surgeon will tell you that such an attitude represents the proverbial "gay abandon of the noncombatant." The administrators themselves are not the ones being exposed, so it is easier for them to advocate that other care-givers expose themselves to danger. We heard of one recent case in which a hospital administrator forced a surgeon to operate on a patient who posed a potential danger, even after every surgeon in the hospital had reached the conclusion that surgery was not indicated, as the patient's life would not be extended. In fact, that patient was operated successfully—the surgeon acting under compulsion—but as all the surgeons had predicted, the patient died of his underlying disease three months later. Fortunately, no one contracted any illness.

So it is easy to stand on the sidelines and tell the surgeon, "Be brave." But let us think it through a little further. When the surgeon makes a decision to go forward, he automatically exposes not only himself but also those other seven or eight important people working in the room to the dangers of contamination. And if the disease is indeed transmitted, what does the surgeon say to his wife? What does he say to his children? Or if his decision results in one of the staff being infected, what does he tell their families? After all, this is often a lethal disease, as I know from sad experience. My own mentor died prematurely at a young age, of hep C contracted in the operating room. He was arguably the most talented, dedicated surgeon with whom I have ever worked. His death affected me powerfully and affects me still.

Especially because of what had befallen my mentor, this issue of hep C was like a raw nerve for me. Of course, I worried for myself, but I worried especially for my family and for the dedicated members of my team.

I told Mr. Minor that I had to consider whether his liver would be strong enough to take the operation without the hep C treatment that he had declined. I also indicated quietly my concerns for myself and my team. I promised Mr. Minor that I would get back to him within three days. I wanted some time to ponder.

In the end, I decided to go forward with the operation. When I did call Mr. Minor several days later to let him know that I had decided to go ahead, I could tell that he was so moved by the decision that he was sobbing tears of joy and gratitude at the other end of the phone line. "Thank you, Doctor," he said, his voice conveying true appreciation. Mr. Minor is such a brilliant and intuitive individual that he had envisioned, I am sure, the debate going on in my mind; being able to understand my concerns, for him, for myself, and for my team, he expressed true heartfelt gratitude at my decision to go forward.

Now it was time to go ahead with the surgery. On April 6, 2006. I performed the operation with the able assistance of my chief resident at that time, Dr. Michael Eng. Michael wrote the most wonderfully complete and detailed operative note, which permits me now to describe the procedure very accurately.

Mr. Minor, being a naturalist with regard to his health, preferred that his bicuspid valve be replaced with a biological valve (that is, one harvested from an animal) rather than a mechanical one. The advantage of a biological valve is that, being made of natural, biological materials, it requires no blood thinners. This is in contradistinction to a mechanical valve, which, presenting unnatural, nonbiological surfaces to the bloodstream, requires lifelong administration of a blood-thinning drug (called Coumadin).

Remember that Mr. Minor had not only a calcified bicuspid aortic valve, but also a large aneurysm that extended all the way down to the heart. Therefore, we needed to replace the valve and aorta as a unit, down to their junction with the heart muscle itself. But biological valves do not come as a prefabricated unit with an aortic graft. (The preservative for the valve is toxic to the graft coating.) So we measured the structures of Mr. Minor's heart carefully by an echocardiogram in the operating room, and then we prefabricated a combination of a valve (sized for Mr. Minor) with a graft (also sized for Mr. Minor), producing what we call a "valved conduit." We did this prefabrication in advance, to save precious time on the heart-lung machine once the heart chambers were open.

We opened the breastbone. We opened the pericardial sac. The aorta was so dilated in diameter and so elongated in length that it had forced the heart to the left side and down toward the belly. The heart normally exerts eminent domain, dominating in its position, but the *aorta*, being so heavily pressurized, can impose its will, even on the *heart*, in terms of command of prime "real estate" in the chest cavity.

We found also that the neighboring heart chambers had moved in toward—and attached themselves intimately to—the root, or lowest portion, of Mr. Minor's aorta. This indicated that the body could tell that the aorta was about to rupture. It was doing its best to seal off the impending rupture by "patching" it with adjacent tissues. Such compensation by the body can mitigate a rupture temporarily, but ultimately the rupture wins.

We put the patient on the heart-lung machine. With the machine taking the place of the heart and lungs, we stilled the heart and opened the defective aorta. We excised the diseased aorta with scissors. We mobilized the right and left coronary arteries, which take off from the original aorta and feed the heart muscle with blood, with a round "button" of surrounding aortic tissues, to facilitate later suturing. (By the way, *Good Housekeeping* magazine got in touch with us after our first report on such use of "coronary artery buttons" in the early 1980s. They thought we were attaching actual sewing buttons to the heart. Once they found out that there were no actual fabric store materials in use, they lost all interest in our work. This all arose because a year or two earlier, some surgeons had closed the abdominal cavity with actual fabric store zippers!)

We next exposed the calcified bicuspid aortic valve. We could clearly see that instead of an opening the size of a quarter or half dollar, the lumen (free channel) had been reduced to the size of a pencil eraser. No wonder Mr. Minor had fatigue. We excised the abnormal valve with a blade and scissors. The leaflets of the aortic valve should normally be soft and supple, like tissue paper. In calcific aortic stenosis, the leaflets are replaced by calcium deposits, as hard and as large as teeth. As we cut and break off these particles, it is imperative to capture each and every piece. Any misstep means a stroke. That is a devastating event for anyone, but it would be especially hard on a man like Mr. Minor, whose mind powers his art, and whose art is his life.

With the defective valve out of the way, we "debrided," or surgically cleansed, the ring of the old valve. We picked out loose pieces of tissue and calcium and then irrigated vigorously with sterile saline—like power-washing with a hose.

At this point, we were in a serious state. We had taken the great normal order of the heart and aorta and induced a state of maximum disorder (entropy). The heart was no longer attached to the aorta. The aorta was no longer attached to the body, which it must supply with blood and oxygen. And the arteries that normally carry the all-vital nutrient blood flow to the heart muscle itself were "hanging in the breeze." All of this anatomy—the heart's normal order (ectropy)—needed to be restored meticulously or life could not continue.

Then, with a series of alternating blue and white sutures, we seated the composite valved conduit (which we had previously constructed) into the ring where the old valve had been. We alternated suture color to make it easier to distinguish the strands of one suture from those of its neighbor.

Next, we delicately burned holes in the main Dacron graft with a microcautery device, to make openings to which we could attach the coronary buttons and their all-important coronary arteries. This attachment process requires meticulous three-dimensional planning—to avoid any stretching, kinking, or torsion (twisting) of the precious coronary arteries. Any irregularity would deprive the heart of blood flow, and the patient would die.

Once the buttons of the right and left coronary arteries were attached, we moved on to attach the end of the Dacron graft to the upper edge of the patient's aorta, where we had cut away the bad aortic tissue.

We were now done with the connections. We opened up the flow of blood to the heart. We let the heart "take a drink" of the pressurized, oxygenated blood—to recover from the deprived state it had been in while on the heart-lung machine.

Now came the moment of truth—the weaning of the patient from the heart-lung machine. We gradually loaded the heart with blood to see if it could take up its normal duty—but Mr. Minor's heart faltered, unable to take over the burden of circulation from the heart-lung machine. This is what every surgeon fears—that after extensive reparative surgery, the heart muscle will not be able to work again. In a case of this magnitude, even a minor irregularity in the way the buttons and coronary arteries lie can produce a situation such as this, wherein the heart is not strong enough to work on its own. That pathway leads to death.

I am sure I took a deep breath. I am sure my blood pressure rose. I am sure I pictured the worst. But we carefully inspected our work. The buttons looked fine. The coronary arteries looked normally full. We started some stimulant medication for the heart muscle, and in a minute, we were breathing easily again. The patient was off the heart-lung machine, his heart muscle beating normally and vigorously. The temporary stumble had been just that—a hiccup in a major cardiac surgical procedure.

We disconnected the tubes from the heart-lung machine. We

closed the chest wall in layers, with heavy wires around the breastbone. We put sterile dressings on the closed wound. The patient was doing very well.

Only then did we find ourselves looking around at one another. The patient was fine. Also, the staff were fine, too: no one had been stuck with a needle, splashed, or spilled on. It appeared we were all safe from the threatening, ugly virions (virus particles) that would gladly have given us hepatitis C.

Knowing Mr. Minor, I am not surprised to note that, because of his awareness of the risks involved in performing surgery on a patient with hep C, he had been very concerned about my safety and that of my team. His first question after coming out of anesthesia was, "Is everyone okay?"

Mr. Minor went on to make an exemplary recovery. Not a hitch was seen. His being trim and very healthy overall paid dividends, permitting him to get up and around quickly. He was home on the fifth day, fully ambulatory.

Mr. Minor sent us a picture of himself and his lovely wife, Florence, "celebrating the one year anniversary of [his] surgery with a walk on the beach in sunny Sarasota." As I write this chapter today, I am struck by their relaxed, carefree aura in that picture, which I have saved to this day.

Wendell Minor has simply excelled in the seven years that have passed since his operation. He has produced no less than twenty additional books in that time, with several more in various stages of completion. I have listed these in a table for you. Please note the distinguished authors who have written the texts for Mr. Minor's picture books, including such luminaries as Buzz Aldrin, Mary Higgins Clark, Robert Burleigh, Jean Craighead George, Ann Turner, and Mr. Wendell's loving and accomplished wife, Florence Minor.

Christmas Tree, *If You Were a Penguin*, and *If You Were a Panda Bear*, if I may be forgiven, are masterpieces representing the collaboration of Florence's writing and Wendell's illustration. Florence and Wendell love to tour schools, libraries, and Head Start facilities to read their works to children—instilling an appreciation of books which, it is hoped, will blossom into a lifelong affair with words and pictures.

Mr. Minor's illustrations have enhanced over two thousand books. Note that number—two thousand—which accounts only for the artwork he has created for book covers. (And unlike so many cover artists, he has dutifully read each and every manuscript, in order to capture the spirit of the book in his cover design.) He wrote and illustrated six picture books of his own and illustrated more than fifty books written by colleagues. In addition to that number, add numerous illustrations for magazines and another thousand-plus illustrations for children's books.

Mr. Minor has won nearly every children's book award in existence, including those from the National Teachers Association, the International Reading Association, the American Library Association, the Parents' Choice Foundation, the Smithsonian Institution, and *Publishers Weekly*, among others. Two of his books were selected for "One Book" Literacy Programs in Pennsylvania and Arizona, and his books are used in classrooms around the country.

Mr. Minor has received over three hundred awards from every major graphics competition. He was awarded silver medals from the Society of Illustrators and the New York Art Directors Club, and gold medals from Creativity International.

A former president of the Society of Illustrators in New York, Mr. Minor has received innumerable honors, in addition to the awards mentioned above. These honors include two honorary degrees, the Ringling College of Art and Design Distinguished Alumnus Award, the Norteheast Children's Literature Collection Distinguished Service Award, and inclusion in the Fox Valley Arts Hall of Fame in Illinois and the Aurora West High Hall of Honor.

Mr. Minor's works have been exhibited widely throughout the country in venues including the Norman Rockwell Museum in Stockbridge, Massachusetts; the Bruce Museum in Greenwich, Connecticut; the Art Institute of Chicago; the New Britain Museum of American Art in Connecticut; and the Boston Public Library, among others. Later this year, the Norman Rockwell Museum will host a retrospective exhibition called "Wendell Minor's America," featuring twenty-five years of his children's book art. A corresponding book featuring the art of the Norman Rockwell exhibit will be published. I have freed my schedule and reserved my lodging to attend that remarkable event.

Pulitzer Prize–winning author, historian, and lecturer David McCullough (who received his undergraduate degree at Yale and, by the way, has won the National Book Award and the Presidential Medal of Freedom) expounds eloquently on the special talent apparent in Mr. Minor's paintings:

Seldom ever in the work of a serious artist is anything there by chance. Sometimes, in a watercolor say, accidents can happen—an unintentionally damp blur perhaps helping to set exactly the mood of a rain cloud—but whether to leave it as is or discard the whole effort and start over is the painter's choice.

It is a point to bear in mind when looking at the work of any artist, but particularly, I think, when looking at a show of the work of my friend Wendell Minor. Everything has been given thought, and as much to what has been left out as to what is included. And this, in combination with his superb draftsmanship, accounts in large measure for the remarkable, characteristic clarity and strength of his paintings.

Painting, like writing, involves considerable thinking—more thinking than most people appreciate—and to paint well, or write well, one has to think clearly, which is hardest of all. "Simplify! Simplify!" is the old tried-and-true art teacher's admonition. Wendell, who worked long and diligently in his student years, learned well the lesson.

Consider his haunting cover painting for Harper Lee's classic novel To Kill a Mockingbird, *a composition that has become so*

*identified with the book that it would be hard to imagine it with
any other cover. The elements are few and simple, each chosen
with a specific intent, each raising its questions, and all rendered
with an almost surreal exactness.*

Mr. McCullough articulates beautifully the qualities that so
impressed me in Mr. Minor's evocative paintings, and which un-
derlie his critical and public success.

Hepatitis C

Hepatitis refers to an infection of the liver, caused by a virus. It
comes as hepatitis A or hepatitis B. Hepatitis A is related to
poor sanitation and is spread person-to-person or via utensils
or contaminated fruit or raw shellfish. Hepatitis B is spread via
blood or body fluids. For decades, it was recognized that there
was another type of hepatitis besides the well-known hepatitis
A and hepatitis B; appropriately, this other suspected disease
entity was called "non-A, non-B hepatitis." In 1989, another virus was discovered as the cause of these other cases of hepatitis, which subsequently became known as hepatitis C. This
virus infects only humans and chimpanzees, but no other species. Hepatitis C is contracted via infected needles, poorly
sterilized surgical or dental instruments, or blood transfusion.

Hepatitis can be asymptomatic—that is, not productive of
any symptoms or feelings of being unwell. However, infections
of long duration can lead to cirrhosis (scarring of the liver),

bleeding from the esophagus due to increased pressure in the liver, or cancer.

There is an effective vaccine for hepatitis B, but none for hepatitis C.

There are powerful (and debilitating) medical treatments for hepatitis C, which can eliminate the virus in selected cases or, in the majority, simply keep the so-called "viral count" down, to prevent late complications. These treatments involve an immune stimulator (alpha interferon) and an antiviral agent (such as ribavirin).

Blood is screened for all forms of hepatitis before being used for transfusion of patients, but screening was not begun in the United States until 1992. Thus Mr. Minor did not have the benefit of blood screening when he had his transfusions in 1964.

If a surgeon or nurse or other health professional incurs an accidental needle stick from a patient with hepatitis C, there is at least a 2 percent chance of contracting the disease. The risk is higher with a deep puncture or if the needle is hollow like a hypodermic rather than solid like a suturing needle.

Monogamous couples usually do not transmit hepatitis C between themselves. Tattoos, especially when performed by unlicensed facilities, can transmit hepatitis C via contaminated needles.

Hepatitis C affects at least 200 million people worldwide, or 3 percent of the world's population.

Many novel treatments for this widespread disease are under investigation, including both vaccines to prevent infection and drugs to combat the virus.

It was my great privilege to be included in the small group of friends and family permitted in the inner sanctum of the huge auditorium where Mr. Minor received an honorary doctoral degree from the University of Connecticut for his extraordinary contributions to contemporary art. (He and Florence recently reminded me that I had to leave a bit early, although not before his degree was conferred and he gave his moving speech, as I had to drive south from Storrs to New Haven to do a heart transplant that Saturday afternoon. I had forgotten that part of the story.) The award of the PhD was especially moving to Mr. Minor, who had grown up before educational science recognized dyslexia, and who had been called and made to feel "stupid" during his formative years.

Boy, did he show them. Today, as I read the transcript of Mr. Minor's UConn address, I sense tears forming in my eyes, hearing of the early life hardships, the return of his father from World War II, the two-room bungalow in which his family lived, and Wendell's love for nature and wide-open spaces and the simple lives and expectations of a Midwestern mid-twentieth-century upbringing. How far this man has taken himself, from his very humble, but exceptionally warm, familial origins.

———

Maryann, our nurse; her husband, Bob; and I had dinner with Wendell and Florence just a few days before this chapter was written, partly so that I could interview them to refresh my memory about his case and his life, and partly just to enjoy an encounter with sheer brilliance. His innate intelligence, his difficult childhood, his brushes with death, his reading and writing, and his lifelong reflections on the human experience have given Mr. Minor unique insights, many of which he extemporaneously and freely shared with us that evening. I have preserved a few of those insightful observations in another information box.

Knowing Mr. Minor has had a strong impact on me. As was the case with other persons described in this book, in getting to know Mr. Minor, I could feel a proximity to greatness. Aside from his talent, the man exudes a calm and a pleasure at being alive, likely forged in his early life challenges as well as his cardiac and surgical experiences.

Those who have died and come back again, if they are introspective and thoughtful, are instilled with a gratitude and appreciation of life. Meeting Mr. Minor also showed me an example of tremendous love for our planet and our environment, and for our natural bodies. Above all, Mr. Minor radiates a special combination of awareness of his talent along with a total lack of conceit. In so many ways beyond his art, Mr. Minor is a model for all of us.

In his own words:

The summer of 1964, between my first and second years at [art school] I was diagnosed with an aortic aneurysm. Emergency open-heart surgery was performed, not once, but twice. I came as close to "buying the farm" as one can. It was a gift, albeit a strange gift, to know at age twenty, that you are on borrowed time, likely for the rest of your life. I've learned never to waste a minute of it. I never have, and I never will!

Reflections by Mr. Wendell Minor

Writers paint with words. I write with pictures.

Dyslexia for me is a gift; it allows me to take ideas from everywhere, from all directions.

I consider creating art for children's books a noble endeavor of the first order.

I approached my surgery in the third person: "Mr. Minor" chose an excellent doctor, so "Mr. Minor" had nothing to fear.

My loves, reflected in my books, are four: History, Science, Nature, Biography.

I did not do well in traditional school systems. My motivation to learn was always simply that I wanted to know, curiosity being my most important virtue. I am committed to lifelong learning.

I taught for eleven years; this was the most valuable training for me. When you teach, you find out what you don't know.

Despite my dyslexia, I have been reading books for forty years. I have done two thousand book covers, and I read each manuscript cover-to-cover, to be certain that I captured the essence of each one.

We think in pictures; that is why movies are represented first in storyboards.

I work in sprints.

I face the fact that some of my work is great, and some is not.

Every book is a child of ours (mine and Florence's).

Florence and I fell in love with Washington, Connecticut, on our first drive through. We were instantly at home. It is a true artists' colony. It is the town that time forgot. It is like a Norman Rockwell painting come to life.

Patience, Passion, and Perseverance are more the secrets to success than innate talent.

Rote is a great tool for memory; we now outsource this to computer applications.

The secret to success is to truly love what you do.

Imagination is built from play: a stick becomes a sword. Kids need to play; they do not need to be encumbered in organized play activities.

One has to treat one's body with respect.

Whom in the creative arts does Mr. Minor most respect?

David McCullough

Pat Conroy

Mary Higgins Clark

James Gurney

Dave Brubeck (he is mesmerized by "Take Five," as am I)

Edward Hopper.

Allow children only limited access to computers before age 7. They need "analog" grounding. The brain is analog.

Chapter 7

Carmella

OUR PATIENTS TEACH US

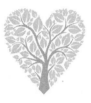

My eyelids open to slits, then shut again. Darkness and light—that's all there is. But the noises are distinctive: machines are busy, sucking and releasing, interspersed with beeps and hissing...

A chemical odor emanates from my throat, like it's coming from a dank cave inside me. Human voices talking around me, muffled. Eyes open momentarily again, then shut. Voices rushing past me, growing louder, then distant. Laughter in the distance. Telephones ringing...

My husband John's voice, talking to someone. Is it my mother? But she lives in Chicago. Eyes open, shut. There are lights directly above my body that are warming me, like a chicken dinner ready to be picked up by the waitress. John and others are talking about my eyes, they are open again. They are sitting around me; they sound hopeful.

I become aware of a huge pipe down my throat, so far down that it seems to create a support for my entire body which, for some reason, is completely limp. I feel the pipe inside me. It seems to go into my chest. I realize that I'm so limp that I'm unable to lift my lungs to breathe. I try to do it. I try to lift my lungs to take in air. I don't have the energy. Will try again later. Thank goodness I have this pipe. I guess it's one of those machines that's breathing for me. I've seen them in the movies. Why is this machine breathing for me? Eyes close.

I hear a voice: "Carmella, can you wiggle your toes for me? Very good, now wiggle your fingers, good, good. Thank you!"

My mouth, face, and neck are paralyzed by the pipe's presence. Chocolate? Eyes open. More voices. "Look, they're open! She must have heard the word chocolate! She always did love chocolate! Chocolate, chocolate, chocolate!" they chant.

A woman is calling my name. Eyes open. How does she know my name? "Carmella, can you hear me?" she asks. I look in her direction. "Tell me your name," she says. Why the hell is she asking my name if she already knows it? What is wrong with her? Eyes close.

A strange nightmare that I can't figure out. Except, every time I fall asleep, I'm also dreaming. Then I keep waking up again to the lights and the pipe. I decide this will be my goal: to figure out which is the dream and which is for real. Eyes close.

Someone is shouting in my ear. "I'm going to take an x-ray. I want you to lie still. It'll be over in a minute."

There are two people pushing me up. A cold metal slab is slid against my back. As they position me upward, the machines come alive with loud beeps and buzzing. The machines disapprove of the movement. Wires are adjusted, the machines quiet down. I'm not only limp, I'm captive as well. Someone has bombed open my chest, there's a giant hole, I can feel it. Won't sitting up make my chest burst open? I sit doubled over, the large pipe down my throat, hissing and pumping next to me. My head, unable to support itself, is flopped forward. My mouth and throat are dry like plaster. The chemical inside me is so strong that I feel metallic, machinelike. If I don't get some water soon, I will die. Don't they know that? Finally, the woman returns, removes the cold slab, and puts me back down.

My eyes open. A nurse is sitting next to me. "Carmella, are you up?" she asks. I stare at her. "Oh, good, let me go get your family." My family? They shuffle in, filing in around my bed. Their mouths are smiling, but their eyes are glassy. They aren't looking at my face. Why aren't they looking at my face? John is the only one who ventures close to me, looking into my eyes and smiling, his face red. He's been crying, I think. I must be unbearable to look at. My own mother can't even look at me. I tell myself I will never react that way toward someone in the hospital if I survive this. Whatever "this" is. Instead, they look down at my body, which is covered up by clean white sheets. There are strange shapes poking from underneath the sheets, though. Mechanical things.

Then a male figure comes in from behind everyone and stands at the foot of the bed. "Uncle Milty is here, Carmella. He's come to see you," John says. Uncle Milty? My father's brother from Chi-

cago? Uncle Milty is the kind of uncle one sees only at weddings and funerals. If there is a major family event, he is sure to be there. Then it hits me: I am dying. I am dying, and my family has flown out here to say good-bye to me. That's why everyone is here. Eyes close.

Someone's hand is holding mine. It is soft, wrinkled, the hand of an old person. Eyes open. "Hello, Carmella, I'm a minister here at the hospital," a woman's voice says delicately. "I'm here to tell you that you are in critical condition." She pauses for a moment. "Carmella, would you like someone to come and pray for you?"

Critical condition? Pray for me? Pray for me? Oh, God, I am dying. This is it. I've wasted my life. I haven't accomplished anything. I'm dying and I'm thirty-two. My father was thirty-four. What about my student loans? Who is going to pay them? Doesn't God care about me? Am I that unimportant to him?

"I'm going to mention some religions, and I want you to squeeze my hand when yours is mentioned," the minister says. "Protestant . . . Catholic . . . Baptist . . . Jewish . . ." I squeezed. Why do they always mention Jewish last? She disappears and, several minutes later, an attractive, well-dressed, twentysomething woman appears by my bed.

Several white coats also appear. The nearest one, who resembles Rod Serling, looks directly into my eyes and speaks.

"My name is Dr. Elefteriades. I'm the surgeon who operated on you." His statement overwhelms me. Somehow I hadn't yet attached a person to all this. I stare at him like he is a long-lost parent. Is this The Twilight Zone? *Is that why I'm so confused?*

He asks me several questions, and gives some instructions to the steadily growing army of nurses standing around him. I am transfixed.

What is his name? Elephant man? Remembering his name becomes another project that occupies my thoughts. Dr. Elefteriades. Elefteriades. Eyes close.

I wake up again. Two white coats are standing on either side of my bed. They are fiddling with the equipment. One of them puts one hand on my head and the other on the large pipe that is down my throat. "Don't move," she says, "we're taking this out."

Slowly, the large tube is extracted from my throat. A gasoline smell comes up with it. I'm a gasoline pump and they're removing the hose. I lie there, my mouth wide open, unable to shut it. I enjoy the fresh air for several seconds, then an oxygen mask is placed over my face and taped down tightly. They fuss with the cords. The machine is pushed away. There is no more hissing, no sucking. Only the sounds of nurses chirping in the distance.

The one who took out the tube turns to me and speaks: "Carmella, we've upgraded your condition from critical to serious. This is very good news." She looks at me with a smile.

Hurray! I'm in serious condition! I take several celebratory breaths through the mask. And I can breathe! I am joyous. I remain joyous. I am still breathing . . . thanks to you.

Written by Carmella Kolman and read by her at the Yale-New Haven Annual Banquet, 2003, describing her experience following her ascending aortic dissection.

As I write this, my wife, Peggy, and I have just returned from a wonderful event. Carmella e-mailed me a few weeks ago to invite me to a small dinner party—to celebrate the twentieth anniversary of her life-saving aortic operation. I was thrilled to accept. It was to be held at the home of Carmella and John's close friends, Dr. Thomas and Colleen Gill, in Westville, a quaint suburb of New Haven, comprising wide, sidewalked boulevards and well-kept, stately, historic houses, located just behind the famous Yale Bowl, where the Yale Bulldogs have played football since the nineteenth century.

We were even more thrilled to arrive and find that Dr. Lawrence Cohen, Carmella's cardiologist, and his "firecracker" wife, Jane, a clinical psychologist, were also in attendance.

And walking through the door, Peggy and I found a radiant Carmella, with beautiful long hair, looking healthy and happy. She wore a dress with a wide, deep neckline, and I noticed immediately that the scar of her median sternotomy had faded almost entirely. I am certain that only I could notice the very faint, thin line of my incision, made so urgently twenty years ago. Cosmetics had been the last thing on my mind as we hastened to open the breastbone, evacuate the pericardial sac of its constricting blood, and control the hemorrhage from the ruptured aorta.

We had a simply spectacular evening, replete with powerful feelings and friendship—as well as phenomenal, thick-cut cod with light breading made by Colleen Gill, a spectacular cook by prior reports and current evidence.

During dessert—ice cream homemade by Carmella—Dr. Cohen asked her to tell us a bit about her background and her journey to her career as an artist.

It was moving to hear a life story whose exact details neither Dr. Cohen nor I had previously known. As we will see, it was the disorder known as Marfan's syndrome that almost took Carmella's life. Now she explained to us that her father also had Marfan's, and it took his life, prematurely, at the age of thirty-four, when Carmella was only six. Her grandfather had died at fifty, also of presumed Marfan's syndrome.

The week before her aortic rupture, Carmella recalled, her beloved dog had been hit by a car. Carmella had lifted the dog, run with him, and felt extreme emotion while rushing him to the veterinarian. We did not know then—though we do now, as a direct result of Carmella's case—that such physical and emotional stress can trigger the initiating internal tear that ultimately results in aortic splitting and rupture. A week later, Carmella suffered excruciating chest pain, as the aortic dissection occurred—the aorta split longitudinally from the heart, around the top of the chest, down the back of the chest, and on to the bottom of her belly. With her family history, she knew she had to call 911, and so she did.

Dr. Cohen was reminiscing on how fate had prepared the circumstances which would permit Carmella's survival. It was a Saturday. It was just after lunchtime. Dr. Cohen was on the hospital grounds, as he had just given a lecture to a group of heart special-ists. So he was instantly available when the emergency room called to say that Carmella was there and that she was in cardiogenic shock. (Carmella reminded him that she had seen him just the week before, and he had told her she would be needing surgery, but that it would be "some time" before it would become neces-sary. Well, Dr. Cohen, joked, "A week is some time, isn't it?")

For me, availability was a bit more of an issue. It was a beauti-ful spring day, and I had the kids. We were browsing the stores around our local Guilford green, my son then four and my daughter seven. My wife was out of town. It was literally the only time I had ever been solely responsible for the kids, so over-whelmingly loaded was my work schedule.

My cell phone rang, and it was Dr. Cohen on the line. Law-rence Cohen is normally a man of few words and of consummate composure. Yet now he was speaking quickly, almost feverishly. "I need you, John. In the ER. Right away. She's dying, John. She's dying right in front of me." When Dr. Cohen called, I jumped, as does everyone else. Now, however, I had a problem: What was I to do with the kids? I had never before faced this difficulty of being needed urgently at the hospital but being solely responsible for my kids. I dropped them hastily, but lovingly, at a neighbor's and was off to the hospital.

In his terse phone conversation, Dr. Cohen had explained Carmella's case. He was particularly distressed because he had been following Carmella's condition for three years, ever since her husband, John Rizzo, had come to teach health care economics at Yale. Carmella was thirty-two years old and had Marfan's syndrome, a connective-tissue disorder that weakens the supportive framework which internally supports the body's organs. It tends to produce aneurysms, or swellings, in the body's central artery, the aorta. Because Carmella's aorta had been only modestly enlarged, Dr. Cohen had not recommended surgery.

Yet this Saturday morning, Carmella had come to the emergency room complaining of severe chest pain. A computed tomographic (CT) scan and an echocardiogram had shown an "acute aortic dissection." This somewhat awkward term refers to an internal splitting of the aortic wall into two layers. Blood under pressure seeps between the layers of the aortic wall and splits them apart, causing the inner layer to separate from the outer layer. The split then propagates all the way down the aorta from the chest into the belly.

Dissection alone can be deadly, as it can result in blocked or diverted blood flow, robbing the heart or other organs of essential oxygen and nutrients. But that was not the worst part of Carmella's story. The scans indicated that Carmella's aorta had ruptured just above the point where it attached to the heart itself. This rupture had released blood into the pericardial sac, the strong membrane that surrounds the heart. The trapped blood, under pressure in the sac, prevented the heart from filling and functioning, sending Carmella into a state of shock. She was drifting in and out of consciousness, her blood pressure was falling, and she was in full-blown cardiogenic shock. In order to survive, she needed urgent surgery.

Having safely deposited the children, I sped to the hospital. Cars are my passion, outside of my work and family; now, in one of my fastest cars, I made the nineteen-mile trip from Guilford to New Haven in about eleven minutes. I figured that, if I were to be stopped by the police, I would have a very valid excuse.

Marfan's syndrome is an inherited disease that weakens the connective tissues in the body, the protein strands that hold our organs together. The aorta is weakened and dilates over time into an aneurysm. Marfan's also affects the eyes, especially the lenses, and Carmella had been born with a severe cataract and strabismus in her left eye. So she explained to us that night at dinner. She had always seen only with her right eye.

She had always loved to draw, back as far as she could remember. Her right eye was impaired by a cataract as well, although it was not as opaque as the one that had damaged her left eye. She remembers holding pictures and photos up close to her right eye as a small child—so that she could see them—and drawing them with pencil and paper.

She had never had three-dimensional vision, seeing only from one eye since birth. Her teachers had told her that her brain had adapted to overcome this limitation, giving her a sense of three dimensions despite receiving only two-dimensional visual input.

Carmella had always been drawn to art. She drew constantly. People brought her projects to draw. When she turned eighteen, she was accepted on a scholarship to the prestigious Rhode Island School of Design, one of the nation's most highly regarded schools of art. She worked hard at college, Carmella told us, but she was a bit of a wild child and she "sowed her wild oats," as she put it.

My sister graduated from the same school, majoring in architecture. We did some figuring, and it turned out that my sister and Carmella had graduated in the very same class.

Carmella taught art for a while, but she was uncomfortable standing and teaching in front of a class. She could tell that the boys were there for the nude models—arriving early and sitting in the front row when a female model was due. Carmella eventually outsmarted them, by deliberately mixing up the dates of the male and the female models.

Carmella eventually gravitated toward drawing and painting professionally on her own. Still lifes became her specialty, first fruit and then flowers.

Doctors had always been afraid to operate on the right-side cataract, worrying that, in case of any mishap to her one functioning eye, Carmella would be incapacitated. Finally, a surgeon agreed to operate. Her cataract was removed—and her vision, for the first time in her life, was normal! She could see that bees had stripes, that ants had legs, and that—horror of horrors—she had fine hairs on her arms and legs. Thereafter, Carmella's vision continued to be normal, although it remained unilateral.

After receiving Dr. Cohen's call, I rushed into the hospital. I met Dr. Cohen and Carmella in the emergency room. Carmella was on the verge of unconsciousness. Her blood pressure was so low—about 80 mmHg systolic—that her brain was not receiving enough blood flow. She drifted in and out of consciousness; when she was awake, she was confused and uttering phrases that made no sense.

"She has ruptured into her heart sac, John," Dr. Cohen told me in his characteristic slow, clear elocution. "You must take her to the operating room immediately."

And that is exactly what I did. My team met me there.

Aortic Dissection

Aortic dissection is an emergency of the highest order. It represents a longitudinal splitting of the aorta into two layers. It is heralded by pain—a knifelike, tearing pain, more severe than any other felt by the human body. Aortic dissection patients who have previously borne a child say the pain of dissection makes childbirth seem like a stroll in the park.

Aortic dissection occurs in the setting of a diseased aorta. The underlying disease can be Marfan's syndrome, as in Carmella's case. Or it may be any of a number of other inherited disorders of the connective tissue—the strands and membranes that hold our tissues and organs together.

Aortic diseases are the fifteenth most common cause of

death of Americans, ranking a little higher than the better appreciated HIV disease in this regard. Even without Marfan's syndrome, aortic aneurysms tend to run in families. Many specific genetic mutations are actively being identified. Dr. Diana Milewicz in Texas has done groundbreaking work in this regard.

Aortic dissection in the ascending portion of the aorta—that is, in the front of the chest, right above where the aorta attaches to the heart muscle itself—is a surgical emergency. Many patients die instantly, without a chance to get to the hospital. The situation looks like—and is often mistaken for—a heart attack. Even among the fortunate few who survive to reach the hospital, without surgery those patients die at a rate of 1 percent per hour, so that a quarter are gone within twenty-four hours, a half within two days, and essentially all are dead after four days. The mode of death is by bleeding into the pericardial sac, a condition called "cardiac tamponade." (See the next information box.)

Emergency surgery can save about 75 percent of patients who have suffered aortic dissection.

Carmella met and married Dr. John Rizzo, the accomplished health economist who has been, from the very day that I met him and Carmella, a cornerstone of our aortic program and the backbone of our investigative work on the natural behavior of the aorta.

Carmella has become more and more prominent in her own work, with art shows at many locations in the country. Despite one-dimensional vision, her paintings have a powerful three-dimensional quality.

Carmella gave us an exceptional still life of fruit—the first painting she did after her urgent aortic surgery. We hung it in our living room. When we lost our house in a fire about four years ago, Carmella's painting miraculously survived, and with some reconditioning, it hangs again on our wall in the new house we built on the original foundation.

Tonight, after her delicious homemade chocolate ice cream, Carmella had yet another surprise for Dr. Cohen and me. She had a still life watercolor for each of us—the colors bright, the dimensions sharp, beautiful to look at. Carmella's is a story of perseverance despite difficulties. She had overcome her eye problems and become, of all things, a painter—a profession predicated on the visual sense. She had handled her Marfan's syndrome with equanimity. When her aorta ruptured and nearly took her life, she recovered, both physically and emotionally, and went on to thrive as a wife and, ultimately, a highly respected artist. Despite the difficulties that life had thrown her way, she has always maintained a positive attitude and a general happiness that are nothing short of remarkable. We see many others with similar challenges who complain and bemoan their fate. Yet here is an exceptional woman who eagerly counts her blessings rather than focusing on the challenges that life has presented.

Carmella is Patient No. 1 in our Yale Aortic Institute Database. Let me tell you how that all came about. As *Scientific American* put it:

> *When a young woman* [Carmella] *nearly died from a ruptured aneurysm,* [Dr. Elefteriades] *and the woman's husband began searching for ways to save other aneurysm patients from catastrophe. The patient had been followed by one of the country's preeminent cardiac specialists—Dr. Lawerence Cohen. Yet, even under his watchful eye, she had dissected and ruptured her aorta. It was clear that medical science needed to study further the issue of when to operate on a dilated aorta to prevent catastrophic dissection and rupture.*

As Carmella was recovering in the hospital after her urgent aortic replacement, her husband, John, and I came to speak more and more fully at her bedside while I was on rounds. John had a PhD in health economics. His specialty was managing and interpreting data, using the most advanced statistical techniques. Now he brought these exceptional skills to bear on the question of aortic diseases. My team and I had vast experience in caring for patients with aortic disease. What, Dr. Rizzo and I speculated, could we accomplish if we combined our skills and talents into an investigative team aimed at better understanding these diseases and improving the criteria for surgical intervention? We thought such a collaborative effort might have merit. Once Carmella was home and recovered, we met formally in my office and embarked on a mission to study aortic disease with the latest, sophisticated statistical techniques, with a special emphasis on predicting when dissection and rupture might be likely to occur. Maybe, we speculated, we could someday write a paper on our findings.

Cardiac Tamponade

The heart is surrounded by a thin, dense, inelastic membrane called the pericardium. The pericardium is probably a remnant bit of anatomy from early on in man's evolution, when it might have provided some protection to the heart from injury by predators.

When there is bleeding from the heart, as from a ruptured aortic dissection, the blood fills the heart sac. Because the heart sac is inelastic and cannot stretch, the accumulating blood compresses the heart chambers themselves. This compression leads to low blood pressure and low cardiac output (forward blood flow from the heart). This quickly leads to shock and, if uncorrected, to death.

In cardiac tamponade, the heart muscle itself is good and strong. The patient lapses into cardiogenic shock because the heart is compressed by the blood in the inelastic pericardial sac—essentially, the heart cannot pump because the heart cannot fill.

The treatment is immediate surgical therapy, with opening of the pericardial sac, to evacuate the blood and relieve the pericardial compression. Of course, the bleeding site itself must also be corrected.

Now it is twenty years later. By applying Dr. Rizzo's statistical analysis to reams of Yale clinical data, we have learned a great deal about the natural behavior of the aorta. We now know, with great accuracy, when the aorta is likely to rupture or dissect. (This happens at about 5 centimeters or more in diameter.) Had we known that twenty years ago, Carmella might have been spared from her rupture event and near death experience. Together, our team has produced over one hundred scientific articles, chapters, and books about aortic diseases. The data accumulated by this team have played a role in developing guidelines for aortic replacement that are applied throughout the world. And all of this began with Carmella's 911 call.

Many discoveries in medicine are accidental, or occasioned by random events. One such event was brought about because of Carmella's Marfan's syndrome and her ruptured aorta. Her personal challenges brought me together with a supremely talented statistical analyst, Dr. John Rizzo. Perhaps this was all chance; I can see that possibility. But once we were brought together by chance, Dr. Rizzo and I did succeed in recognizing that our collaboration would provide an opportunity to advance medical science. A few years ago, I was asked to give an important address as part of a formal "Leadership in Bio-Medicine" lecture series. My address had two themes. The first was "Our patients teach us." That was certainly true in Carmella's case. The second was "Fortune favors the prepared." That was true of Carmella's story as well: once we had met, under the circumstances that brought us together, Dr. Rizzo and I recognized that our fields of knowledge could mesh in a way that would extend medicine's knowledge of aortic diseases.

Thus, Carmella's is a story of personal human spirit and triumph, but also one that illustrates how important it can be to take advantage of an apparent serendipity when life is really handing an opportunity.

Carmella's eloquent, moving, emotional description of her awakening from anesthesia after her life-threatening aortic rupture and urgent corrective surgery testifies to her vivid sense of her environment—which I am sure is a factor in her ability to convey beauty and emotion so well in her paintings.

I think of Carmella, with gratitude, every time I look at that painting of fruit that hangs on my living room wall.

The "Sandwich Technique" for Aortic Dissection

In an aortic dissection, the aorta splits into two layers—an inner and an outer layer. These are thin layers. The mid-portion of the dissected aorta must be resected—that is, cut out—but the artificial aorta needs to be sewn to the dissected aorta at each end.

Now when the aorta is dissected, the aorta to which one sews the graft is like wet tissue paper. One always worries that it will not hold the stitches. To combat this tissue weakness, we make a "sandwich" of the dissected layers. We put a strip of Teflon felt inside the aorta, and a strip outside the aorta, sandwiching the weak tissues in-between. The felt on the inside and the outside prevents the stitches from tearing through, giving us a better chance of making an attachment that will hold without tearing and bleeding. This whole process requires judgment, delicacy, and experience.

Chapter

8 | Robert Norton

MEMORIES

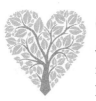 Of all the students in my class at Lansdowne-Aldan High School in Lansdowne, Pennsylvania, back in 1968, one sticks out in my memory.

His name was Wayne, and he was bright and pleasant and humorous. But he didn't have many opportunities to demonstrate those traits, because Wayne had what we call in medicine an "unusual facies." In layman's terms, he was "different looking."

Wayne was tall, exceptionally so, and gangly. I would estimate that he was nearly seven feet in height. His arms and legs were very, very long, and he was rail thin, with no muscle or fat on his limbs or his torso. He wore thick glasses. Classmates shied away from him.

Despite these challenges, Wayne did well in school. He maintained a very small, but close circle of friends, and he matriculated to a local college.

Shortly after we graduated from high school, word went around that Wayne had died in a car accident. He was the very first among our classmates to die. I was deeply saddened and have remained affected by his death to this day. I remember that his favorite song was "House of the Rising Sun" by The Animals. Although I love that group's music, whenever that particular song comes on the radio, I have to shut it off. I cannot hear it without being reminded of Wayne's untimely and unwarranted death.

Had I known back in high school what I know now, I would have recognized immediately that Wayne had Marfan's syndrome, like Carmella in Chapter 7. His condition would have made him particularly vulnerable to the huge physical forces that can come into play in an automobile accident. Even a minor collision could have been enough to tear his presumably enlarged, thinned, and weakened aorta. He must have died instantly.

But this is not a story about Wayne. This is a story about Robert Norton, another name that brings a tear to the corner of my eye.

When I was called urgently to the Pediatric Intensive Care Unit on September 5, 1991, the first thing I noticed about Robert was how closely he resembled Wayne. He, too, was a tall, thin, teenage boy. He had been transferred from Danbury Hospital, about forty miles to the west and north of Yale. Danbury is an upscale community, close enough to New York to qualify as one of its suburbs. The accomplished cardiologist Dr. Samuel Felder examined Robert there and made the diagnosis of Marfan's syndrome with acute aortic dissection.

My former colleague, the distinguished Dr. Charles Kleinman, one of the nation's preeminent pediatric cardiologists (and years later my surgical patient), put it succinctly in his letter:

Robert is a 15 year old young man with Marfan's syndrome who presented with a catastrophic aortic dissection from the aortic root, around the aortic arch, into the great arterial branches, and down the descending aorta to the iliacs, with involvement of the renal and superior mesenteric arteries.

In other words, Robert's aorta split into two layers (see Chapter 7, page 162), a phenomenon called aortic dissection. The split had involved his entire aorta, from the vessel's origin at the heart, around the top of the "candy cane," and all the way down to the bottom of the belly. The dissection had sheared off multiple important branches in the process, including those to the brain and the intestines.

Marfan's syndrome, which weakens the aorta and other structural tissues throughout the human body, is hereditary, and Robert's family history bore this out. Robert's mother, Ruth, forty years of age in 1991, carried the diagnosis of Marfan's syndrome. She had evidence of weak "connective tissues" within her body, manifested in multiple ways. Four years earlier, she had a spontaneous pneumothorax; that means that her lung ruptured on its own, releasing air into a pocket around the lung—a dangerous condition requiring placement of a tube to drain the air. The pneumothorax was able to occur because the lung tissue was not as strong as it should have been. She suffered also a dislocation of her jawbone two years previously—again, because the ligaments of the joint were not as strong as they should have been. And Ruth had mitral valve prolapse, reflecting a weakness of the connecting "cords" that normally prevent excess movement of the leaflets of the valve. However, unlike Robert, Ruth's aorta was of normal size.

Ruth's father was very tall and very thin, like Robert, and he died suddenly following a hernia repair at the relatively young age of forty-nine. Hernias are characteristic of Marfan's syndrome, reflecting weakness of the fascia—the membranes that line the body cavities. Sudden death in Ruth's father likely represented a dissection with rupture, just like Robert himself presented to us when I was called to the Pediatric ICU.

Robert's father, though very tall at six-foot-six, was not thought to have Marfan's syndrome. And my patient's two younger brothers, while tall like their father, did not show any signs of Marfan's.

Of note, Ruth's sister had also been diagnosed with Marfan's. Her aorta was severely enlarged (60 millimeters, whereas normal is up to 38 millimeters). Surgery had been recommended for her aorta. Her twenty-two-year-old son was diagnosed with Marfan's, too.

The Norton family demonstrated vividly the protean manifestations of Marfan's syndrome, and the fact that it is transmitted in what geneticists call a "dominant" family pattern, so that half the offspring get the gene and everyone who gets the gene develops the disease. However, not all patients inheriting the dominant gene develop the full disease (what we call "incomplete penetrance"), so those who do inherit the gene can have widely varying manifestations in different organ systems.

Dr. Kleinman and his team stabilized Robert in the Pediatric ICU overnight, and we took him to the operating room early the following morning. Also caring for Robert was the highly regarded pediatric intensivist (a specialist in serious child health care problems) Dr. George Lister.

When we opened the breastbone, we could see the severely enlarged aorta even through the pericardium, the sac around the heart. The pericardium itself was discolored, evidence that blood had leaked from the aorta into the pericardial space. We opened the pericardium, revealing a black, enlarged, irritated aorta—a very bad dissection. The enlargement of the aorta went all the way down to the heart, meaning that we could not "simply" replace the aorta (although that is *not* a simple task); rather, we needed to perform an even more extensive procedure. We needed to replace everything, right down to the heart, including the aortic valve and the coronary arteries.

At the top end as well, we needed to do extensive surgery. We had to put Robert into suspended animation by cooling him to a very low temperature and shutting off the heart-lung machine in order to effect a complete removal of enlarged aortic tissue at the top of the aorta. We accomplished this with Robert in suspended animation for thirty-four minutes. But the tissues were so weak that bleeding occurred after we finished the repair, and we had to open the aorta a second time to place reinforcing sutures in those very weak tissues. This is a serious turn of events. Many patients die after an emergency operation for aortic dissection, often from bleeding. Ultimately, in Robert's case, with the re-opening of the aorta and internal reinforcement of our suture lines, we were successful in controlling the bleeding. Robert stabilized after this huge, lengthy surgical procedure. He was transferred in stable condition to the Pediatric Intensive Care Unit. Recognizing the extreme underlying tissue fragility, I said at the conclusion of my operative report, "Short and long term prognosis will remain guarded."

The operation was ultimately successful. Miraculously, despite the fact that two brain arteries and one intestinal artery had been sheared by the original dissection, Robert woke up intact, and his brain and intestines were fine. After our repair, the blood directed itself properly into those sheared arteries.

Eventually, after several days in the ICU, Robert was stable enough to be transferred to a regular pediatric floor.

I got to know Robert and his fine family a bit during the days he stayed on the pediatric floor completing his recovery. Every inch of the walls of his room was covered by his artwork, some brought from home, and some created by Robert from his hospital bed during his recovery. I remember an abstract quality to Robert's paintings, and what I can only call an *intensity*.

Robert always had something to tell me during my visits, in an animated way, with energy. His conversations were not the usual that would be expected from a teenager. He tended toward the abstract and the obscure—like a savant.

I thoroughly enjoyed my visits with Robert. I had a sense that Robert was in some way "on a higher plane" than the rest of us. Also, I thought of my former classmate, Wayne, who had lived and died in a time when the surgical therapy to repair his condition had not yet been developed.

Robert continued to improve. He did require drainage of some fluid that accumulated around the heart—done by a needle aspiration—but his recovery was otherwise uneventful, and he was discharged to go home with his parents.

I personally breathed a sigh of relief that this young man, so special, so reminiscent of my deceased classmate, had survived in good condition and gone home. The entire pediatric and surgery teams were thrilled. Victory was at hand.

Robert was able to return to school full-time. An aid was assigned to help him carry heavy books and to prevent him from being injured in crowded hallways.

Dr. Kleinman and I were very happy when we saw Robert in follow-up that October and December.

There was, however, one red flag raised during the December visit. You will remember that the entire aorta had been dissected—the layers split from the heart to the bottom of the belly. As always, we had replaced only the six inches of aorta between the heart and the top of the chest. This is standard. The remainder of the dissected aorta normally "heals" itself, in the sense that the outer layer of the aorta thickens and strengthens.

But this favorable healing is not always the case with Marfan's patients. You will remember that Robert's aorta had been especially fragile when sutured in the operating room. Inspected under a microscope, the specimen of diseased aorta that we removed showed advanced weakening of the aortic wall. In fact, where layer upon layer of strong connective tissue should have been located, Robert had microscopic lakes of fluid. The connective tissues had been destroyed by Marfan's syndrome.

Talented, Creative Celebrities with Aortic Aneurysm Disease

Robert Norton, as you can see, was very creative. I have had so many extremely creative patients with ascending aortic aneurysms that I have begun to think that the mutation that causes the aneurysm to occur, as in Marfan's syndrome, may confer increased creativity as part of the spectrum. Think of all the especially creative individuals felled by aneurysm disease. Albert Einstein died of aneurysm disease. Lucille Ball, the iconic comedic actress, died of an ascending aortic dissection. Jonathan Larson, the author of *Rent*, never saw his play open because he died of ascending aortic dissection the night before its Broadway debut. He had gone to two New York emergency rooms, but he was thought to be too young and healthy to have heart disease, and he died after being discharged from both. His play opened the very next day. The respected dramatic actor George C. Scott died of aneurysm disease. The beloved John Ritter, of *Three's Company* fame, died of ascending aortic dissection, having been misdiagnosed as suffering from a heart attack. And of course, Carmella Kolman, the subject of Chapter 7, falls in the category of exceptional creativity.

My distinguished teacher, Dr. M. David Tilson, a leading aneurysm researcher, gave a credible talk at one of our aortic symposia—upon my challenge—arguing that there is indeed scientific evidence for a connection between aneurysm disease and a creative mind. Some scientific studies have suggested emotional and intellectual differences in Marfan or other aneurysm patients compared to the general population.

In December, we discovered that the aorta in Robert's abdomen had started to enlarge. This part of the aorta had been normal in size—about 1.5 centimeters in diameter—when the operation was done in October. By December, it was 6.0 centimeters—an extremely rapid increase, at almost unheard-of speed. We referred Robert for examination by Dr. Richard Gusberg, a superb clinician and an expert in the abdominal aorta. We were especially concerned because Robert complained of back pain, and the location of the pain corresponded to the area where the aorta was growing rapidly.

By February, the abdominal aorta was 10 centimeters in diameter! The aorta could not grow much more without catastrophic rupture. Something needed to be done. Robert needed an operation lower down in the aorta, but that posed an added level of complexity and risk. There was a 20 percent or more chance that surgery would leave him with permanent paralysis of the legs.

Once we understood how rapidly Robert's abdominal aorta was growing, I met with him and his parents. I explained (quoted here from my visit note), "It has now become clear that the descending thoracic and abdominal aortas have grown at an alarming rate. The infrarenal abdominal aorta is about 10 centimeters or more in largest dimension." I could clearly feel the enlarged abdominal aorta when examining Robert's abdomen. I explained to the family that "it is not prudent to delay any further in embarking on an operation . . . [because] . . . rupture can be expected given the dimension of his aorta at this time." I emphasized the severe danger of the operation to replace the remaining aorta: "I made it abundantly clear to Mr. and Mrs. Norton that Robert's case represents a very, very serious problem which will be difficult to manage even with the experience that our teams in cardiac surgery and peripheral vascular surgery have with such problems."

I was thinking ahead and further explained to the family that we would need to replace the entire remaining thoracic and abdominal aortic segments—everything remaining of the aorta, in other words. I further explained (from my visit note), "This is an operation of the greatest magnitude. It may not be possible to obtain control of bleeding during such an operation, as we very well may be limited by the quality of the dissecting tissues." I was remembering in my mind the extreme fragility noted at the first operation, as well as the severe destruction of the aortic wall by Marfan's syndrome seen under the microscope in the specimen of aorta that we had removed at the first operation. My notes from the consultation said, "I emphasized the possibility of death from operation and made it clear that there is a significant likelihood of its occurrence."

We took Robert, now sixteen, to the operating room on February 19, 1992. The most recent MRI scan had measured the aorta at 13.5 centimeters. It was expanding more rapidly than any aorta I have ever seen, before or since.

We opened through a long incision running from the top of the back, across the chest, into the abdomen, and down to the pelvis—what we call a thoracoabdominal incision.

We worked for hours and hours. Every stitch tore the fragile tissue. For every suture line, innumerable extra stitches had to be placed. Dr. Gusberg and I, along with our teams, and with the anesthesiologist, Dr. Charles Kopriva, toiled incessantly. I am stubborn. Dr. Gusberg is stubborn. We do not take no for an answer. We would not stop in our efforts to save this boy. We placed stitch after stitch. We used trick after trick and maneuver after maneuver, calling on all our experience, resolve, and reserve.

But hours and hours, and all our abilities, were just not enough. You may imagine how I felt, later that day, when I dictated these words: "It was not possible despite maximum medical measures to maintain hemostasis (control of bleeding), and vital signs (pulse and blood pressure) deteriorated and the patient expired."

Dr. Gusberg and I went home that night exhausted and demoralized. We had not wanted to permit the death of that special young man. I had gotten close to Robert over the months since his life was first saved, and I had developed a strong sense that he was different from the rest of us. He was special, and I believe surpassed us in many ways. I could not accept the mortal outcome of our efforts. Also, I am sure that Robert's death resonated in my subconscious mind with the death of my similarly afflicted classmate, Wayne.

When I finally went to bed with my wife that night, I cried. The sadness simply overwhelmed me once the trappings of everyday life yielded to the privacy of the bed. I was embarrassed to have my wife hear me cry, but she knows me well, she understood, and she com-

forted me. I had not shed tears in many, many years, but I cried that night.

We had saved this patient when he presented with his virulent ascending aortic dissection. We could not save him when, a number of months later, the abdominal aorta dilated ferociously. My disappointment that Robert Norton could not be saved has been a motivating factor in my career-long research to better understand virulent aortic diseases.

We did obtain a postmortem examination on Robert, hoping to learn more about his case and his Marfan's syndrome. The postmortem showed that Robert's brain was substantially larger than normal, a full 2 kilograms—one-third larger than normal. Furthermore, Robert's brain showed complete congenital absence of the corpus callosum. The corpus callosum is a wide, flat bundle of nerve tracts; its 250 million individual fibers connect the left and the right hemispheres of the brain, permitting intercommunication between the two sides of the brain. So Robert's brain was indeed special—large, with the two hemispheres separated and not in normal communication.

In terms of Robert's aorta, the microscopic examination found the abdominal aorta "degenerative" and "necrotic"—in other words, the wall was so badly affected by Marfan's syndrome that it had been destroyed and had died. Poor Robert's aorta had been genetically programmed to destroy itself at a very young age.

Did Lincoln Have Marfan's Syndrome?

Historians have become interested in whether the great American President Abraham Lincoln had Marfan's syndrome. He certainly was tall and lanky like Marfan's patients. Why do historians care? Well, with ascending aortic aneurysm, the aortic valve may leak as the aorta dilates, its leaflets being distracted (pulled apart) until there is a gap in the middle, like the flippers of a pinball machine. The leaky valve increases the difference between the systolic blood pressure (the upper number, as the 120 in 120/80) and the diastolic blood pressure (the lower number, as the 80 in 120/80). This makes the pulsation of your blood vessels more prominent. If it gets really bad, you may be able to see your pulse beating in your fingertips. If it gets very, very bad, your limbs themselves may "bob" with each heartbeat.

Historians have concluded that, in a famous photograph, Lincoln's left foot was bobbing. They further surmised that the bobbing was due to a leaky aortic valve, that the aortic valve was leaking due to an ascending aortic aneurysm, and that Lincoln therefore had Marfan's syndrome. Now why do historians care? Well, without surgical therapy—which Lincoln certainly could not have had in the nineteenth century—very few Marfan's patients survive beyond the mid to late forties. So presumably Lincoln would have died soon anyway, even if he had not been shot at Ford's Theatre in 1865.

Chapter

9 | Bill Vinovich

THE REFEREE

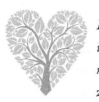 *It is Saturday, January 12, 2013, and I am watching the AFC Divisional Playoff Game. It is Baltimore Colts at Denver Broncos. The temperature is zero degrees Fahrenheit and the elevation is one mile high, so the air is thin and cold. I am enjoying the football, but I am keeping an eye on the chief referee, William "Bill" Vinovich. For reasons that will become clear as you read this chapter, I am worried about the referee in this supremely inhospitable environment. The cold is dangerous to him, as is the altitude.*

Out on the field, emotions are running high. There have been controversies. So much rides on this game. It will determine which team goes to the Super Bowl. I am holding my breath, hoping and praying for this game to be over. I want to see the ref walk out of the cold back

into the warmth of the locker room. I want to know that he is safely back on an airplane headed to his warm, sea level, hospitable place of residence, Orange County, California.

It is an exciting game. My prayers for a quick end to the game are not answered. Baltimore ties the score with less than a minute to play. The game goes into overtime. I cringe, picturing in my mind the strain put on the referee's aorta by the exertion, the intensity, the emotion, and the altitude.

Enough already! Can't this game end? But no, now we are into another overtime. The announcer informs us that this is now the fourth longest game in NFL history.

My blood pressure is, I am sure, running high. "How can this be?" I ask my wife. "Why does Bill have to have such a long game, under such adverse circumstances? I want this game over."

Finally, Baltimore wins on a field goal. I breathe a sigh of relief. Bill looks well. He doesn't even look cold. He doesn't look tired. I realize that he is doing what he lives for, what he is meant to do. He is completely at home and in his element as an NFL referee, regardless of the hostile physical and meteorological environment.

Anyway, the game is over. I stop worrying. I am responsible, after all, as you will see.

Dr. Jeffrey Borer is an exceptional cardiologist. In fact, word has it that he was designated as the best cardiologist in the state of New York. He is among that very rare breed of physicians who are both world-class clinicians and world-class researchers. He is also among the vanishingly rare breed of physicians who are extremely capable and confident, yet modest, self-deprecating, and unassuming. You can tell from this description how much I respect Dr. Borer. I admire him even more because of his background in athletics. He was a discus thrower in his youth, and one can still see the impact of the athletics from his bearing and silhouette.

Dr. Borer has been the cardiologist for the NASA program as well as for the National Football League. Periodically he calls on me to see an athlete with aneurysm disease, to assist in difficult decisions about permitting or not permitting continued participation in athletic activities. Whether to allow an athlete to compete or to bar him from participation is an overwhelmingly important decision for the athlete—both emotionally and financially.

Dr. Borer called me about Bill Vinovich, and my life was enriched by that call and by coming to know Mr. Vinovich and his family.

Dr. Borer was worried about Mr. Vinovich and felt he probably should never return to his position as NFL referee. Mr. Vinovich was very upset and wanted to explore every possibility. "Please look at him and let me know what you think," Dr. Borer requested.

Athletics can be dangerous for patients with aneurysms. Please see the information boxes.

After an introductory phone call from Dr. Borer, Mr. Vinovich flew out from California to Connecticut to see me. I remember when he walked into my office for an afternoon consultation, after I had finished my work in the operating room.

He was at once a commanding presence (six-foot-two and 215 pounds), but at the same time he radiated a personal warmth and kindness toward others. The office staff had already whispered to me that they were quite taken with him. He carried himself very gracefully, like a natural athlete. He sat back in the chair in front of my desk in an ankle-over-knee position that bespoke confidence and authority. He came in by himself, he explained, as his wife and kids were back on the West Coast.

He was fifty years old. His status as an NFL chief referee, he explained, made him one of a very small fraternity. He had played wide receiver at Santa Ana College and the University of San Diego, but he was not destined to play professional football. He became a referee, and that, he said, other than his family, was his life. He loved his job—the excitement, the challenge, the high stakes. He wanted to referee again. Without that opportunity, there was a huge void in his life. I noted in my medical report from his first visit to my office: "He is absolutely devoted to his career, more than life itself, it appears from this interaction with him. It means everything to him to get back to his work as an NFL referee, both emotionally and financially."

Mr. Vinovich explained that, in 2006, he had suffered an acute aortic dissection—a splitting apart of the aortic wall layers—of the descending aorta. As is standard with dissections in that location, he was treated without an operation, with medications alone, to keep his blood pressure very well controlled.

Good blood pressure control discourages growth or rupture of the dissected aorta.

The dissection had occurred while Mr. Vinovich was lifting weights—just like the case with the young man in our information box. (Mr. Vinovich explained that in college, when he was six-two and 185 pounds, he used to bench-press 320 pounds. At his current age, he was using much smaller weights when the dissection occurred.) The high blood pressure brought on by the weight lifting had split the aorta into two layers. Fortunately, the aorta had not ruptured externally, and Mr. Vinovich survived after being treated with medications that lowered his blood pressure and decreased the strain on the aorta—but no operation.

Mr. Vinovich had survived and recovered. But a dissection never goes away—the patient always lives with a "double barrel" aorta, although the aorta does scar and thicken as it recovers, decreasing the chance of early rupture. Over time, an aorta that has suffered an aortic dissection does enlarge progressively and ultimately may rupture, especially if it is put under strain from high blood pressure or severe emotion or extreme exertion. Many patients with such a dissection will eventually require surgical intervention.

Ever since he suffered the dissection, the National Football League's executives had not permitted Mr. Vinovich back on the field, for fear that the physical exertion and emotional stress could put his life in jeopardy. They had consulted Dr. Borer, who shared the concerns of the NFL and who, in turn, requested my opinion.

Mr. Vinovich had returned to refereeing for college basketball, but he wanted to referee again in the NFL. To do so was of immense importance to him. He told me that, if I could clear him to get back on the NFL field, neither he nor his family would hold me responsible in any way in case of any adverse event on the field. He would sign papers to this effect, he emphasized.

Interestingly, Mr. Vinovich is a fully trained certified public accountant, and he has always practiced accounting during the "dark period" for referees—between the Super Bowl in February and May 15, when preparations for the new season begin. (That explained the facility with numbers that Mr. Vinovich manifested in all our interactions.) Note, please, the favorable correspondence between the NFL "dark period" and the height of the tax season, peaking on April 15. One would not normally associate the skills and personality traits of an NFL referee with those of a certified public accountant. I found this range of abilities in Mr. Vinovich intriguing, adding another dimension to his persona.

At the time of his office visit, I examined Mr. Vinovich. His physical exam was normal—he was to all external appearances a healthy, fit, relatively young man. But his external appearance belied what was going on internally within his chest.

We looked at the studies that Mr. Vinovich had brought with him. The CXR was quite abnormal. We could see that the descending aorta, where the dissection had occurred, was enlarged and bulging to the patient's left. Furthermore, the ascending aorta could be seen bulging to the right. This was a different zone of the aorta to that which had dissected a number of years earlier. The CT scan confirmed what the CXR indicated.

I certainly shared Dr. Borer's concerns about letting Mr. Vinovich return to the playing field. I said in my consultation letter: "I believe that the exertion and emotion of such a charged environment [the NFL football field] could potentially be detrimental. I have explained this to the patient. He is anxious to find some way that I can give him clearance to participate, including offering to sign a waiver releasing me of any responsibility in case of adverse event. He indicates that he has discussed this fully with his family and that they are in agreement. He has traveled today alone from California for the purpose of today's visit."

Mr. Vinovich's view was very clear: He wanted to ref again. He pointed out, to give me an additional push in the direction he wanted me to go, that he made much more salary refereeing just a few NFL games per year than he was making currently doing many, many college basketball games.

Once again, Mr. Vinovich explained, he would not hold me in any way responsible in case of an adverse event.

I told Mr. Vinovich that I needed to reflect on his situation. Would the presumed leathery scarring of the descending aorta be enough to keep him safe in that region? What about the enlarged ascending aorta? I was concerned that it could split under the physical and emotional strain of the gridiron. Should we remove that portion surgically at this point in time? Would doing so make me comfortable enough to allow him back on the field?

I asked Mr. Vinovich to go on back to California and call me in one week. I have cared for literally thousands upon thousands of patients with aortic problems of all kinds, and I have almost never needed to delay giving my opinion. But this was a situation I wanted to study and consider further. I also wanted to "sleep on it," because I have found that letting my unconscious mind deliberate on a difficult issue helps me clarify the best course to be taken. The more experience I get, the more convinced I become that our instinctive intelligence is more powerful than our conscious intelligence. Scientific studies have backed up this notion—essentially that our "gut" is smarter than our brain. Our new president of Yale University, Peter Salovey, is, in fact, one of the world's authorities on emotional intelligence.

Most patients do not call when we tell them to call. Patients tend toward procrastination and denial. But one week to the day after our visit, Lorena buzzed in on my phone: "Mr. Vinovich—the referee—is on the phone for you." I had studied his case in my mind subliminally, and I had formulated a plan, which I shared now with my patient over the phone.

I explained the following to Mr. Vinovich. I was not too worried about the old dissection in the descending aorta. The diameter had been stable, at just under 5 centimeters since early after the dissection occurred. I knew from voluminous experience operating on these aortas that the outer layer of the descending aorta had probably turned "leathery" by now, likely providing some protection from rupture, even on the football field.

I was more concerned, I explained, about the ascending aorta, which was also just under 5 centimeters in diameter. It was the ascending aorta that tended to dissect in the young athletes in our clinical experience and in our scientific analysis and writings.

The ascending aorta was an especially vulnerable portion of the aortic anatomy.

So what I offered for Mr. Vinovich's consideration was the following: We operate to replace the ascending aorta and the aortic arch, the part carrying the arteries to the brain and arms. After successful completion of such surgery and full recovery, I indicated to the ref, I would be willing to clear him to return to the gridiron.

This was surgery of the greatest magnitude, I explained. There were substantial dangers involved: death, stroke, and bleeding, among others.

"You will let me referee after you have completed this operation?" Mr. Vinovich asked, wanting complete clarity.

"Yes," I answered.

"Let's do it. How soon can we schedule it?" was the referee's response.

He was not deterred by the magnitude of the operation or the risks involved. "I know you will bring me out fine, Doc," he added before we finished our phone conversation. "Thank you very much for your decision."

So Mr. Vinovich came out to Yale in June 2011, this time with his family. Dr. Cleman, our premier catheterizing cardiologist, did the obligatory coronary angiogram, which showed that Bill had no significant coronary artery disease despite some underlying high cholesterol.

I went up to my patient's hospital room to see him the night before the scheduled operation. There I found the nicest family one could ever want to meet. His wife, Jeanette, a senior manager at Disneyland, was as sweet as could be. The young son was respectful and quiet, worried for his father. The young daughter was just as beautiful as her mother, and as worried as her brother.

I reviewed the situation fully for the family, reiterating what I had covered in my separate sessions with Bill. I gave the information, including the risks, but emphasized the positives. When I left the room and walked down the hallway, I found myself feeling under even more pressure, now that I had met that model family. This compounded my concerns—about Mr. Vinovich himself, about the fact that he was Dr. Borer's patient, and about his high profile in the NFL.

Strength Training and Aortic Dissection

A number of years ago, our aortic nurse specialist, Maryann Tranquilli, pulled on my shirtsleeve as we were making rounds in the ICU. We were about to round on a twenty-eight-year-old schoolteacher with no history of cardiac disease who had come in a few days previously with an ascending aortic dissection. "Doc," Maryann said, "why have we had all these young athletes with aortic dissection?" She had noticed a pattern to which I had paid no attention. "We have had three healthy athletes come in with aortic dissections in the past eighteen months," she reminded me. "Why is that?"

I replied that I did not know, but that we would get to

the bottom of it. Maryann reviewed our records, and she found a total of five young athletes—two more than even she remembered—all with ascending aortic dissection—all occurring during weight lifting.

We had identified a phenomenon that we did not understand. I could not answer Maryann's insightful question about why aortic dissection was befalling these young men. So we went to the laboratory—in this case my home gym—to investigate. My son, at that time a healthy sixteen-year-old athlete, did the investigation as his tenth grade science project. Together with our talented anesthesiologists, Dr. David Silverman and Dr. Robert Stout, we fashioned a device that could measure the blood pressure instant-by-instant during weight-lifting maneuvers. We did the experiment on ourselves, so that we did not need to explain to Yale's Human Investigation Committee why we were subjecting volunteers to an activity we felt was precipitating aortic dissection in our patients.

Remember that a normal blood pressure is 120/80. My son raised his blood pressure to 180 mmHg while bench-pressing 100 percent of his body weight. I myself have been lifting weights since I started my wrestling career at age thirteen. I raised my blood pressure to 220 mmHg while bench-pressing 100 percent of my body weight, 178 pounds. We had to stop our anesthesia colleague, as he reached a blood pressure of 320 mmHg bench-pressing only 75 percent of his body weight. These are astronomical elevations of blood pressure during weight lifting—not seen in any other environment or situation, not in the surgical ICU or in the medical ICU. Professional weight lifters, we found, can reach 380 mmHg during their lifts.

My son got only a C on his science project—his teacher did not like the study—but he was able to get the paper published in *JAMA* (one of the world's most prestigious medical journals)! Go figure.

After we published that first paper, we had reports sent to us from around the country, and we amassed nearly three dozen similar cases of aortic dissection in athletes engaged in vigorous strength training.

Of note, all these individuals had underlying aortic aneurysms, of which they were not previously aware. Weight lifting became the lynchpin, raising blood pressure at the instant of the lift above what the diseased aorta could tolerate.

Still, I slept fine that night. Years earlier, I would toss and turn the night before a dangerous, difficult, or especially high-profile case. About a decade ago, the realization sank in that very few individuals had as much experience with the aorta as I had amassed. As well, I had come to understand that there was never any question of my needing to care more deeply or try harder surgically for any patient. So from these realizations, I derived a sense of calm. I could not guarantee a positive outcome for any specific patient, but I would bring to the table all the experience, willpower, caring, and determination humanly possible.

It was seven thirty the next morning, and I made my way into the operating room. Patty, the senior circulating nurse and an aortic specialist, greeted me at the door. "He is a good-looking man, John, and in great shape." Mr. Vinovich had made quite an impression on the nursing staff, not only by his appearance but also via his personal charm and warmth. "He will do fine," Patty added. I respected her judgment and appreciated her encouraging words. Administrators these days often fail to understand the importance of the teamwork, camaraderie, and mutual respect that develop within a specialty team in the operating room. Arbitrarily assigning unfamiliar personnel, however well accredited, as current exigencies often require, is not without detriment.

Mr. Vinovich later told me that he was not scared at all going in for the operation. He cited two reasons. First, he had checked out the credentials of our team fully. Second, to get everything done in time for the next season, all the preparations had been made very quickly, "and I simply did not have enough time to get scared," he explained.

By the time of my arrival in the operating room, Dr. Gerald McCloskey had put Mr. Vinovich to sleep and placed all the invasive monitoring lines. He did an ECHO exam via a probe he placed down Mr. Vinovich's esophagus, the swallowing tube. Such an ECHO exam provides crystal-clear images, because of the physical proximity of the esophagus to the heart itself. Dr. McCloskey confirmed the dissection in the descending aorta and the enlargement of the ascending aorta. The heart muscle itself was good and strong.

A Father's Story

I am sharing with you a phone call I received after we published my son's paper on the link between weight lifting and aortic dissection. We received calls and letters from many parts of the United States. I found a number of these calls simply heartbreaking. I share one story with you.

A hospital president called from New Jersey. Now hospital presidents are of necessity tough and hardened. This gentleman cried for one hour as he spoke on the phone with me. My heart went out to him. This was for him a very painful phone call—profoundly so—yet he wanted me to have the information, to help others in the future.

Tearfully, he told me the following story:

His son was a twenty-one-year-old junior at an Ivy League school. He was a football player. His team had played on Saturday (and won). This young man was so dedicated that he was in the university gym at 8 a.m. the following morning, even though the team had the day off, doing a weight-training workout so that he could be a stronger and better football player.

He had been doing bench presses with large amounts of weights. He stopped his workout and went to the infirmary because he had developed pain in his chest. The staff in the infirmary saw before them a healthy, athletic, muscular young man—too young and healthy to have heart disease, they felt. They called his father to tell him he did not need to come. The young man had strained his pectoral muscles, they explained.

What stands out in retrospect is that the young man told

everyone he saw—the secretary, the triage nurse, the clinical nurse, and the doctor—that he was dying.

By 6 p.m., someone thought to get an ECHO of the heart. The ECHO was done, and it showed a dissection of his ascending aorta, with rupture into the pericardial space (the heart sac). The heart was squeezed by the surrounding blood and consequently unable to pump blood. The patient had lapsed into cardiogenic shock from cardiac tamponade. (See Chapter 7.)

A helicopter was called to take the young man to the nearest major medical center, but he was dead before the helicopter arrived.

The father's tears are understandable. What is extraordinary is the father's putting himself through the pain of relaying this heart-wrenching story. He did this because he wanted to support our efforts to understand this phenomenon that takes the lives of young athletes. He wanted his son's data included. This, I felt as I listened to the father's tearful tale, is a man who truly cares about his fellow man.

We embarked on a huge aortic operation. My assistant was my chief resident, Dr. Chris Terrien, as fine a human being and as talented a surgeon as I could possibly wish for. We opened the breastbone, and we could see the ascending aorta bulging against the pericardium, the heart sac. When we opened the pericardium, we could see that the ascending aorta was large and "angry." By this I mean that it was red and had irritated markings on its surface—like the conjunctiva of your eye when you get a particle stuck under your eyelid. Furthermore, the aorta was very fragile, suggesting a weakness of the aortic tissue from birth.

Our first job was to find a place to hook up to the heart-lung machine. We exposed and cannulated (put a bypass tube into) the axillary artery, the artery that exits under the collarbone and supplies blood to the arm. But that cannula did not bleed back properly. That was an inauspicious beginning, as safe attachment to the heart-lung machine is a *sine qua non* for a successful outcome. Our fallback position was to put the tube from the heart-lung machine directly into the diseased ascending aorta, not a very palatable thought. But given no more attractive alternatives, that was exactly what we did.

We went on the heart-lung machine, fortunately without adverse consequences. We stopped the heart, and we cut Mr. Vinovich's aorta just above the coronary arteries, the arteries that supply blood flow to the heart muscle itself. We sewed in a Dacron graft that was 24 millimeters (1 inch) in diameter. This went well.

But the aneurysm extended up higher. We had to cut more and go up and detach the arteries to Mr. Vinovich's brain. We call these arteries the innominate artery and the carotid artery. For this phase of the operation, we had to put Mr. Vinovich into suspended animation. We cooled him to a very deeply cold level (18°C, or 64°F), so that his brain would not require much blood flow or oxygen supply. Then we stopped the heart-lung machine completely. Mr. Vinovich was now entirely without any blood flow. His blood pressure was zero. His EKG (heart wave) was flat. His EEG (brain wave) was flat. The heart was at a standstill. In this state of real-life suspended animation, the patient's state is indistinguishable from dead.

We now turned our attention to the aortic arch, the "candy cane–shaped" top of the aorta. We cut the arteries to the brain right off the aortic arch, so they were "hanging in the breeze." We then cut out the aortic arch itself.

Now, during deep hypothermic arrest, the technical name for the deep-cooled suspended animation, the clock is always ticking. The requisite repairs must be completed in forty-five (or at most sixty) minutes or brain damage will occur.

We sewed a graft into the remaining dissected aorta in the back of the chest, a long reach from the incision in the breastbone. This occupied twenty-five minutes. We pulled back an extension of this graft, like unrolling a sock. To this extension, we had to connect the brain arteries. We worked diligently at this task, and all the while the clock was ticking.

In many operating rooms, the time while the patient is in deep hypothermic circulatory arrest is one of high tension, frayed nerves, and barked orders. In our room, because we do this nearly every day, we have a relaxed environment. Although the whole team is totally focused—and my world and that of my assistant are reduced to the one square foot of open chest in front of us— we concentrate without undue anxiety or acting-out behaviors.

We sewed and sewed, and the head vessels were attached. We brought this part of the procedure home in a very safe total of forty-one minutes.

We resumed flow from the heart-lung machine while we made some secondary graft connections and rewarmed the patient.

Have you ever had Greek egg-lemon soup? It is a delicious chicken soup made with a touch of lemon and a touch of egg. The best Greek cooks know that, to avoid curdling of the egg droplets, they must patiently simmer the soup very slowly. Otherwise the egg droplets will curdle and spoil the appearance and flavor of the broth. With mild simmering, the egg dissolves entirely, with no curdling or particles visible.

Now why have I taken us out of the OR and into a Greek kitchen while we were in the middle of this huge operation? Because the egg white is made of a protein called albumin, as mentioned in Chapter 3. Mr. Vinovich's bloodstream, like yours and mine, was full of albumin. And if we rushed his rewarming on the heart-lung machine, his albumin would have curdled (denaturing of the protein). This would have resulted in a bloodstream full of "scrambled eggs." This would have been extraordinarily dangerous, sending off particles to the brain, heart, and other organs, resulting in stroke, heart attack, and other devastating internal injuries.

So we always warm slowly. We never heat more than 10°C above the current temperature of the blood.

We successfully warmed Mr. Vinovich. His heart started to beat. Then came another moment of truth. We needed to "wean" him from the heart-lung machine—to see if, after this very extensive surgery, the heart was strong enough to beat on its own and handle the burden of circulating the blood.

Mr. Vinovich's heart took the load easily. His heart maintained an excellent blood pressure. Dr. McCloskey's ECHO exam showed vigorous contraction of the pumping chambers of the heart.

The great many "hookups" we had sewn seemed intact and dry.

We breathed a sigh of relief and closed Mr. Vinovich's chest.

We transported him back to the ICU. I walked with my team during the transport process, never straying more than a few feet from Mr. Vinovich at any time. I breathed another sigh of relief upon safe arrival in the ICU.

But I did not like what I was seeing. The vital signs were all fine, but there was excess drainage from the chest tubes, the large-bore, garden hose–like tubes that we leave under the breastbone to evacuate the obligatory blood and fluid that are liberated by the operated tissues.

We like to see less than 100 cc of drainage per hour. Mr. Vinovich's blood pressure had been high since our arrival in the ICU, and he had already drained over 600 cc in less than one hour. With so many hookups, so many sutured structures, the elevated blood pressure may have encouraged a specific spot to start to bleed.

Now when I am concerned, I do not shout and blame. Rather, I turn quiet. My repartee with the staff I have come to love dearly ceases. The nurses and residents can read me like a book. I was quiet now, not happy with the picture that I was seeing.

I called the OR to let them know we needed to return for a "reexploration"—a "look-see."

Please reflect on what the surgeon feels in such a circumstance. Things may turn out fine. Reexploration is not uncommon, especially after an operation of this magnitude—maybe one in twenty cases. But what if the bleeding causes shock or tamponade before we get to the OR? What if the bleeding is from the farthest anastomosis (hookup) and we cannot reach it?

And, of course, I am thinking to myself, *This man is only fifty. He has that lovely family. He has two kids, the same genders and ages as mine—the very same. And he is high profile—he is an NFL chief ref, after all. And above and beyond that, he is a patient of Dr. Borer's. I cannot let anything happen to him.*

The cardiac surgeon always worries about death. It can happen. It can easily happen in operations of this magnitude. It can happen in situations just like this, when there is excess ongoing bleeding. You can imagine what the surgeon's blood pressure does in such a circumstance. No surgeon wants any patient to die. That goes without saying. But it is different for those patients who have achieved extremely advanced age and have only a year or two to live under the best of circumstances. Surgeons most hate to lose children or young adults. A vigorous, relatively young, distinguished, vibrant family man like Mr. Vinovich falls in the category that one would most hate to lose.

I had felt a special bond with Mr. Vinovich from the moment

I met him. We were not too far apart in age. Although he was an excellent athlete and I a mediocre one, athletics had always been and continued to be an important part of my life. Our families were of parallel structure. He had achieved the highest distinction in his chosen field through hard work and dedication, and I also had certainly worked hard and been dedicated to my career.

So on many different levels, I did not want this man to die.

When the going gets tough, I have several mechanisms on which I call.

During my training, I had experienced a number of different patterns and styles with which my surgical teachers responded to serious or desperate situations—many by loud denigration and blame of others on the team. I taught myself early on to take a different posture. First of all, I get very quiet because I am thinking— thinking hard to find a way out of the problem at hand. Second, I never blame anyone but myself. Third, I suppress any emotion. Early on, I taught myself to be the "ice man": the harder the going gets, the more composed and concentrated I become. This has stood me in good stead throughout my career.

Finally, I do not hesitate to pray, usually silently, asking God to help me find a way to help my patient in need. Perhaps the dearest of the many, many thoughtful presents I have been given by patients is a watercolor painting that shows a surgical team working diligently in a patient's chest. If one looks closely in the background, one sees the faint outline of Jesus, and his hand is gently resting underneath the surgeon's elbow, guiding his right hand. This is how I feel about any talents I may have in my profession—that they are skills and talents given to me to help others. When I pray, I ask for such guidance. I had that watercolor, in the vinyl standing cover in which it came, on the bookcase next to my desk in my home office. I found it especially and consistently very moving.

We lost our home in a fire about five years ago. It was very difficult, more so for my wife than for me. The fire started next to my home office, in which I had the watercolor I just described. The room was completely destroyed by the fire, having been at the epicenter of the flames and the prime target for the water hoses and demolition applied by the wonderful firemen who responded. When we were able to enter the rubble that was left, the vinyl frame of that watercolor had survived. The painting itself was gone, but the frame had enough identifying information to permit my reordering the watercolor, which is back on my desk in our new house, which we rebuilt on the original foundation.

As we wheeled Mr. Vinovich back toward the operating room for bleeding, to reexplore his chest cavity, I became the ice man, and I said a quick prayer for guidance en route.

Postoperative bleeding was much less common before the FDA withdrew a powerful drug called aprotinin, which prevented many of the deleterious effects of the heart-lung machine on the clotting components of the blood. This withdrawal of aprotinin from the market is now being questioned, and many experts have come to feel that one particular physician overstated the complications of this drug. Aprotinin is being reconsidered for return to the market in a number of countries, including the United States.

A different drug, called Factor VII, is now sometimes used for patients with bleeding after cardiac surgery. Factor VII reverses some of the deleterious effects of cardiopulmonary bypass on the clotting elements in the blood. Factor VII is definitely dangerous, however, and much more so than aprotinin had been. With some trepidation, we administered a small dose of Factor VII to Mr. Vinovich before we headed back to the operating room.

Mr. Vinovich was still sedated and on the breathing machine. I do not believe he was at all aware of the bleeding and the return to the OR.

On arrival in the operating room, Mr. Vinovich appeared quite stable. We used powerful intravenous medications to bring his blood pressure down from the high levels it had reached. Bringing down high blood pressure is always good for the control of bleeding, because it lowers the pressure head feeding any bleeding sites. Also, it appeared as if the blood was becoming thicker, possibly reflecting the beneficial action of the Factor VII.

We replaced the ECHO probe, and the heart looked fine, with good strong function and no blood accumulated in the pericardial sac. The bleeding from the chest drains subsided. We watched in the operating room for two hours, and the situation appeared to have resolved. We did not need to reoperate.

We returned to the ICU, and from there on, Mr. Vinovich progressed properly and quickly. He awoke beautifully, and his breathing tube was removed later that evening. I went home late that night, finally confident that we were back on course. By morning, Mr. Vinovich was out of bed and took a walk. His strength, fitness, and exercise background paid dividends, as he recovered very quickly and his lungs worked exceptionally well. He continued to be very popular with the nurses, his charisma and good humor always in evidence.

The ref was discharged to the suites owned by the hospital, where he stayed with his family. He continued to recover well, taking walks around the Yale campus with his wife and children.

But two new problems came up about a week later. First, the patient developed a rapid heartbeat, called "atrial fibrillation," which is exceptionally common after cardiac surgery, affecting 30 to 40 percent of all cardiac surgical patients. This made him feel a bit uncomfortable and a little short of breath. As well, due to the blood thinners required, he developed what we call a "pericardial effusion"—a collection of fluid around the heart. This added to the shortness of breath.

So, a week post-op, we went into the operating room again. We made a tiny incision between the ribs and let out about a quart of watery fluid from the pericardial sac. At the same sitting, we also delivered an electrical shock to terminate the atrial fibrillation and restore what we call "normal sinus rhythm."

Two days later, Mr. Vinovich was back at the suites with his family.

A week after that, my wife and I had lunch with Mr. Vinovich and his lovely wife, Jeanette. He was so strong and healthy that one could no longer tell that he had undergone recent extremely extensive cardiac surgery. During our lunch, we enjoyed learning more about Bill and Jeanette. They had met at college, where he was a football star and she a cheerleader. It was like a story from a movie script. Where do you take a couple from Orange County, California, where physically beautiful surroundings abound? Peggy took us on a tour of the Connecticut shoreline communities, and then we went to the Stone House Restaurant, right on the water in scenic Guilford. Even our Angelino guests found the setting beautiful. We talked a lot about our families and our children. It became clear that Billy, as his wife called him, and Jeanette were devoted parents and just the nicest people one could ever hope to meet. Bill's love of football was always in evidence, but despite his important position, he was truly and genuinely a modest man.

Mr. Vinovich continued to do well after his return to California. His health continued fine. I wrote a letter to the NFL indicating my permission for him to return to the gridiron. I knew his new Dacron ascending aorta could take the strain, and I was betting that the originally dissected descending aorta had become leathery enough to keep itself safe under stress. Dr. Borer endorsed the clearance to return, and the NFL ultimately granted permission. Bill was back to his passion—again a referee in the NFL.

Bill's return to the gridiron was the Detroit at Philadelphia game on October 14, 2012. I watched that and Bill's other games on TV whenever I could, and I felt proud to know him—his character and intelligence and ability and integrity prominently in evidence in his conduct on the field. I enjoyed his decision pronouncements for the camera, where his confidence and unparalleled knowledge of the game were in full evidence. I was secure in having permitted his return to the field, but I will admit that I wanted that playoff game (from the start of this chapter) conducted in overtime, zero-degree weather to end. Stress and cold and prolonged exposure represent just about the maximum challenge an aorta can face—a perfect storm, of sorts. Finally, the game ended, and I breathed easy again.

Today, as I am writing this chapter, I have received an e-mail from Bill. He addressed it to Maryann, our incredible aortic nurse specialist; to Lorena and Jodi, who run the office; and to Carol and Jenna, two nurses from the floor. It is the second anniversary of his operation, which was done on June 21, 2011. Here is what he wrote:

Hello All!

I just wanted to touch base and say hi and Thank You all again for all your tremendous care and support.

Today is my Two Year Anniversary from the date of my surgery.

As you know, I was able to return to the field last season because of all your great talents! It was sincerely a dream come true. I was just notified that I will have my own Crew this season. Hopefully, I will make it to New England or New York and stop by to visit.

Thank you all again! Stay Well! Hope to see you all soon.

Very Truly Yours.
Bill

———————

Bill is universally loved. While I was watching coverage of the San Francisco versus Seattle Sunday Night Game, I saw Bill charge angrily toward the camera. He had just broken up an on-field altercation after a play in which a player was knocked to the ground *after the whistle had sounded.* Bill looked genuinely angry. The commentator, Al Michaels, speculated that Bill was about to eject a player. Instead, Bill issued a foul for "player activity"—manifesting the judgment, wisdom, experience, and restraint that have earned him a stellar reputation. Said Mr. Michaels:

> *Bill Vinovich, the Referee. Before he makes the call—It's good to see Bill back. He was a Ref in 2006, then had major surgery, an aortic aneurysm, had to have it removed, then went to the league office and finally gets cleared again.*

On the NBC show *Pro Football Talk*, the panel spoke about Bill Vinovich's return to the game of football. The panel and Jim Daopoulos, a former referee himself, had the following to say:

> **Eric Kuselias:** *It seems like every week the officials take a hit. They take an awful lot of abuse. And they are easy to hit for fans. But there*

is a really nice story this week among the officials. Can you tell us something else about that?

Jim Daopoulos: *Sure. In 2006, one of our Referees, Bill Vinovich, was taken off the field because of a medical issue. He worked with me up in New York. He was the Supervisor, the West Coast Supervisor of officials. And he did a great job. Yesterday, in the Detroit—Philadelphia game, he was back on the field for the first time, and it was great to see number 52. He will bring a lot of integrity. He will, Eric, bring some experience. He is just a good official and exactly what they needed out there. It is great to have Vinnie back out there.*

The panel of that show sure got it right. Talent. Commitment. Experience. Integrity. Those words describe Bill Vinovich perfectly.

Bill recently told me an anecdote of which I was not previously aware. He reminded me that he had atrial fibrillation after surgery, when he was up on the regular floor. Nurse Carol had just finished her shift and was doing her charting. Nurse Jenna came on duty.

As Bill stated it, "Jenna came on that evening and started her normal examination, listening to my heart, abdomen, and intestines."

She said, "Oh, it sounds so gurgly."

Bill's son, Billy, then asked Jenna, "What does it sound like? Does it sound like a whale? I speak whale." He was mimicking a line from the movie *Finding Nemo*, where a character named Dory the blue fish (voiced by Ellen DeGeneres) thinks she can "speak whale."

Billy continued imitating the character, sending Mr. Vinovich into a fit of laughter that he could not stop, even though it was causing him excruciating pain in his chest incision.

His daughter, Shawna, held a pillow to her dad's chest. "You're going to kill Dad!" she shouted at Billy.

Just then, the alarms went off: Flatline! Mr. Vinovich's heart had literally stopped from the effects of the uncontrollable laughter.

Jenna was composed. "It will come back," she said. "Just wait."

And so it did. And better yet, when the heartbeat came back, the atrial fibrillation had stopped, and Mr. Vinovich was now in normal sinus rhythm. The laughter had stopped his heart, but also favorably converted the rhythm. Maybe *Reader's Digest* is right: that, at least sometimes, laughter really is the best medicine.

We had an opportunity for Bill to tell me a bit more about the AFL Divisional Playoff Game in Denver with which I started this chapter. He was not aware, he explained, of the specific dangers related to the cold. He did point out that it was indeed very, very cold on the field that day. At the start of the game, he already had on two shirts, yet he had to run in and put on a third shirt to stave off the cold. He never uses gloves during a game, but on that day, he gave a pair of gloves to an assistant on the sidelines—to have them ready, just in case. As the game wore on, he realized that he did indeed need them. He went to put them on at halftime. (NFL halftime, unlike college halftime, is only thirteen minutes, Bill reminded me.) Trying to put on the gloves during halftime, he quickly realized that it was so cold that his hands had swollen and the gloves no longer fit. He simply couldn't get them on.

"Now I know how OJ did it," he added wryly in describing the events to me.

You may not know this, but referees are graded and rated for every play of every game. Bill was proud to tell me that his ratings were good enough for him to be selected to work the Divisional Playoff Game that was discussed above. Furthermore, his scores were so good that, in his first year back, he was selected as an alternate referee for the Super Bowl. He was there at the 2013 game in New Orleans when the lights went out!

He recently let me know that he has been assigned his own crew of officials for next season. (The officials for a game, he explained, are seven in all: an umpire, a line judge, a head linesman, a side judge, a field judge, a back judge, and the referee.) With his typical modesty, Bill offhandedly revealed that he is on the short list for referee for Super Bowl XLVIII in 2014.

So this chapter is about an exceptional man with a great family. He absolutely loves his work. He excels at his work. He showed great cour-

age in undergoing extensive surgery, both to preserve his safety from his aneurysm disease, and to permit his return to football. One only needs to watch him referee, to see the keen, quick decisions he makes in high-tension, on-field controversial plays and calls, to realize that the deep hypothermic arrest protected his brain very well, as our studies have shown. The ref, Mr. Vinovich, enhances people's lives not only on the field, but in every environment, through his love of life, his love of sports, and his personal charisma and warmth.

I Am On a Mission

Now that we know what causes aortic dissection in these young athletes, we can take measures to prevent the senseless loss of these promising young lives.

Our studies showed that an acute rise in blood pressure during weight lifting was the inciting factor for the aortic dissection in the young athletes. But, it turned out, all the affected athletes had underlying aortic aneurysms about which they were unaware. Without the underlying aneurysm, nothing would have occurred. Only in the presence of an enlarged aorta, our engineering studies showed, did the tension in the wall of the aorta rise high enough to split the wall and produce an aortic dissection. For those of us without an aneurysm, we can lift to our heart's content.

So the issue becomes to detect aneurysms in athletes. This can be done by ECHO. The Olympic Committee no longer allows any athlete to compete in the Olympic Games without a cardiac ECHO. (The ECHO can detect not only aortic aneurysm, but also a handful of other conditions that can put the heart at risk.)

My mission is to implement routine cardiac ECHO examinations for all college athletes who participate in heavy strength training or exceptionally rigorous sports such as football or wrestling. Our team at Yale, led by the cardiologists Dr. Sandip Mukherjee and Dr. Jaime Gerber, has developed what we call the "snapshot" ECHO exam. This is a focused ECHO exam (much quicker and simpler than a full ECHO) which can rule out aneurysm and all the other abnormalities that can threaten the heart of a young athlete. The exam is simplified so that it can be performed by a team trainer. It can then be read in minutes by a trained cardiologist. We feel we can keep the cost below $150.

Now the realists say, "John, do you comprehend the social and financial implications of your recommendation for routine ECHO exams?" Yes, my critics are right. Millions of ECHO exams would be required. And exercise-related aortic dissection is a rare phenomenon. My recommendation is not fiscally justifiable, my critics say.

But those critics did not hear the hospital president's anguished call. They did not hear the dozens of other stories of bereaved parents, siblings, spouses, and children. And after all, a pair of Nike shoes for the athlete costs up to $500. Let's just do the $150 ECHO and save these young, promising, dedicated, disciplined lives.

Chapter

10 | Pete Kenyon

THE OLYMPIAN

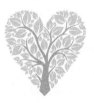 A dedicated athlete stands on the block, about to begin the 200-meter freestyle race at the 2008 U.S. Transplant Games. This extraordinary swimmer—a gentle man with a many-faceted professional background—is about to win a gold medal in this race, setting a new U.S. Transplant Games record in the 60 to 69 age group. That is exceptional in its own right, but even more exceptional is that he will swim and win a gold medal *with someone else's heart* beating in his chest.

Pete Kenyon has competed multiple times in the World Transplant Games, winning four gold medals and setting four World Transplant Games records in the four freestyle events (50, 100, 200, and 400 meters). He has competed in seven World

Games and won thirteen medals in all. I will tell you more about this man, about his critical illness, about his will to live, and about the manner in which he appreciates life and lives it to the fullest—extracting all the challenge, human interaction, satisfaction, and essence that each and every day has to offer.

Mr. Kenyon's background remains a bit obscure. I have known him, and participated in his care, for more than a decade and a half—but a shroud of mystery still persists. He has been involved in many types of activities—as you will see—and rumors about his exciting past have probably embellished the already very real excitement of his early adult life. I will concentrate on what I know to be fact.

Mr. Kenyon has been a competitive swimmer since his youth, participating and winning in local, regional, and national swimming meets. Although he did not compete in high school, he was a varsity swimmer his freshman and sophomore years in college, focusing on the butterfly and freestyle events.

Mr. Kenyon knows that I love cars—always have, always will—and he has told me several times about his association with the great race driver of the 1970s Peter Revson. Many older readers will remember Peter Revson as the handsome, charismatic playboy—heir to the Revlon fortune—who happened to be a superb Formula One and Indianapolis 500 race driver. Mr. Kenyon, I believe, served as the trackside mechanic for Revson for several years at the beginning of Revson's racing career. So race car mechanic is another hat that Mr. Kenyon has worn.

Mr. Kenyon is a former Navy surface warfare officer, who

retired as a commander. He served on a destroyer and made two deployments to the Western Pacific Fleet [WESTPAC] during the Vietnam era. Destroyer activity in WESTPAC included plane guarding, which consists of following an aircraft carrier during flight operations in case a pilot needs to ditch his airplane. This plane guarding task requires maneuvering among a number of larger ships at a fast tempo, an acute tactical awareness, and very quick situational analysis to permit proper maneuvering decisions; all are essential in order to avoid being hit by "one of the big boys."

Mr. Kenyon was recruited for an all-volunteer mentoring program, helping young men prepare for Naval Special Warfare training (SEALs, SWCCs, EOD Techs, Navy Divers, and Air/Sea Rescue Jumpers). Since he had volunteered for UDT (Underwater Demolition Teams—the legendary "Frogmen") while he was in original Navy training—but was not selected due to a high school knee injury—this new mentoring opportunity was gratefully and enthusiastically accepted! He is now the executive officer of the program.

When I ask about what he does now, Mr. Kenyon explains that he is in the reinsurance business—insuring insurance companies, to be specific. I then ask him, What does all that jargon mean? It means, he explains, that the reinsurer underwrites bulk portfolios of insurance policies issued by other companies. Hopefully, the underwriter selects wisely and makes a profit in these transactions. It becomes clear that Mr. Kenyon has to be smart, with a real knack for numbers, and keen analytical skills, in order to ascertain which policies merit his buying—and which ones can turn him a profit over time. As you will see, Mr. Kenyon's clear mind, his way with numbers, and his analytical skills were all brought into play a bit later in his life, and those abilities guided him through the difficult life-and-death decisions that he had to make when his heart failed him.

<hr />

Mr. Kenyon was sixty years old when I met him in 1998. He had suffered two heart attacks at fifty years of age, which had left him with what we call "ischemic cardiomyopathy." *Ischemia* is a Greek word meaning insufficient blood flow. *Cardio* is a Greek word for heart. And *myopathy* is a Greek word for muscle weakness. (As you can garner, my Greek heritage helped me tremendously in getting through medical school.) So Mr. Kenyon had a weak heart due to insufficient blood flow. Usually, such heart attacks are caused by arteriosclerosis, hardening of the arteries. In Mr. Kenyon's case, however, it was not arteriosclerosis, but rather a congenital kinking of an artery that had led to the blocked blood vessel and, subsequently, to the heart attacks, which had ravaged his heart muscle, eventually critically.

As often happens, the large heart attack zones led to dangerous arrhythmias, or runs of irregular heartbeats. On New Year's Eve in 1990, Mr. Kenyon received an implanted AICD (automatic implantable cardioverter defibrillator, a mechanical device that automatically shocks a bad rhythm when it occurs), as increasingly stronger drug therapy was not working to control his irregular heart rhythms. With this device implanted and working well, Mr. Kenyon was able to return to work, even commuting into downtown New York City two or three days a week from Darien, Connecticut.

With his heart failing and the future bleak, it was decided that Mr. Kenyon's only chance for survival was to replace his heart with an artificial organ. His condition was too precarious for him to wait the months or years that it can take for a suitable donor heart to become available. He needed an instant replacement for his heart—one that could be taken off a shelf—and that left only the option of a mechanical heart. But in 1998, dealing in mechanical hearts meant sailing in relatively uncharted waters.

On August 11, 1998, my colleague Dr. George Tellides— both an excellent clinical surgeon and a superb molecular biological scientist—and I took Mr. Kenyon to the operating room to implant an accessory mechanical heart.

Mr. Kenyon had already had one heart operation, and that meant reentry into his chest was quite dangerous. As you will recall, after a first operation, the body no longer has glistening, smooth internal membranes. Rather, once the irritative insult of a surgical procedure has been imposed on a body cavity, that cavity will no longer have clean, pristine anatomy. Instead, the operated-on surfaces stick together, one membrane adhering to another. In the case of open-heart surgery, the heart muscle itself can adhere to the inner table of the breastbone, making reentry exceedingly dangerous. The saw used for reentry can, simply put, cut into the heart muscle itself.

Artificial Hearts

You have probably heard of Robert Jarvik, whose work with the total artificial heart is listed among the top 100 accomplishments of the twentieth century. Dr. Jarvik trained as a physician, but he applied his brilliant intellect to pioneer the development of artificial heart devices. This entire field came to the world's attention in 1982, when Dr. William DeVries (the surgeon) implanted a Jarvik 7 artificial heart in patient Barney Clark at the University of Utah. Remarkably, Mr. Clark survived for an amazing 112 days.

Since those early days, efforts became redirected from the development of total artificial hearts, replacing the function of both the right and the left ventricles, toward the more modest, but more achievable, goal of replacing only the important, muscular left ventricle—the one that pumps blood to the whole body.

In the 1980s, these devices were very bulky, consisting of actual bellows-like pumping chambers. The Novacor and HeartMate pumps competed against each other just as the Chevy 327 V-8 car engine competed with the Ford 289 V-8 in that very same era.

Then Dr. Jarvik, with another stroke of genius, developed a miniaturized pump, about the diameter of a Cuban cigar (but half the length), which propelled blood not via a bellows, but rather by a miniature fanlike impeller. Since that time, other manufacturers have developed their own devices, also operating on the fanlike impeller principle. These smaller devices are much easier to implant than the device that we installed in Mr. Kenyon.

Artificial heart technology has advanced considerably over the last three decades. Not only are devices smaller, but they are less likely to produce clots and emboli (which can cause heart attack or stroke). In fact, the technology is advancing so rapidly that it has now become a close call whether a patient would want a heart transplant or take his chances with a permanent artificial heart device.

In this case, we used an oscillating saw on the breastbone, one designed to cut the stiff bone but—we hoped—able to spare the soft, vulnerable, vital heart muscle. We got through the bone safely. As always, we breathed a sigh of relief at that milestone.

We went on to create a large pocket for the artificial heart device in the plane below the abdominal muscles but just in front of the peritoneal sac, the membrane containing the internal abdominal organs. The Novacor device that we hoped to implant—which our team at Yale had used since its first clinical trial—was very large—about the size of a drinking canteen. It could not be accommodated in the pericardial space itself or in the chest cavity; only the abdomen was large enough to accommodate this mechanical behemoth.

Having created the pocket, we went on to dissect the heart from its surrounding structures. The pericardium had stuck to the heart muscle, and the heart muscle had stuck to the lung—all as a reaction to the prior surgery. Here the going got tough. Mr. Kenyon's severely diseased heart was very sensitive, and each time we gently pushed it aside to divide the adhesions—the connecting tissue bands formed by the reaction to the prior surgery—Mr. Kenyon went into VT, or ventricular tachycardia, the abnormal heart rhythm you see on TV that is treated by shocking paddles. The external paddles were not able to correct Mr. Kenyon's VT, and due to the adhesions, we had no room to place the internal paddles. We were in a very serious situation—with the heart in a terrible rhythm which could not generate a pulse or blood pressure—and no way to convert that rhythm electrically. We had no choice but to quickly connect Mr. Kenyon to the heart-lung machine, which we had in readiness, to support his heart during the remaining dissection of his pericardial space.

That done, with the safety margin provided by the heart-lung machine, we went on to dissect out the remainder of Mr. Kenyon's heart from the adhesions.

We now attended to the business of implanting the artificial heart and connecting it to Mr. Kenyon's own heart and blood vessels. We put stitches all around the heart muscle at the apex of the left ventricle. Remember from Chapter 1 that muscle itself is very weak for suturing, so this process is always precarious. We excised a core of muscle from the apex of the heart—removing a piece about the size of a black beaker stopper from chemistry class. Through that opening, we placed the large connector that would channel blood to the Novacor. Then we connected a large, cloth ouflow tubing from the Novacor to Mr. Kenyon's ascending aorta. That tubing would ultimately carry fresh, pressurized blood from the Novacor to all of Mr. Kenyon's organs.

These connections made, we came to the moment of truth. Would the connections hold, or would they bleed in a life-threatening or even life-ending fashion? Would the Novacor work properly, and be able to carry the load of circulating Mr. Kenyon's blood?

We gently turned down the heart-lung machine and turned on the Novacor—weaning from the former and transferring load to the latter. This did not go well. Mr. Kenyon's own heart, which still needed to beat to supply blood to the lungs, again manifested its irritability, going once more into ventricular tachycardia. We had to reinstitute cardiopulmonary bypass, shifting the load entirely back to the heart-lung machine.

We administered powerful cardiac-stimulating agents intravenously and again began the weaning process. Again the Novacor mechanical heart failed to support the circulation adequately. Mr. Kenyon once again lapsed into VT.

On close inspection, we could see that, as invariably happens to some extent, some air bubbles had been entrained into the bloodstream, and that was hurting the native heart. (Air in the arteries causes a "vapor lock," preventing nourishing blood from reaching the hungry heart muscle.) We de-aired again and again.

Two unsuccessful attempts at weaning from the heart-lung machine boded poorly. Dr. Tellides and I were both concerned. The unspoken communication between us was tacit and intuitive.

Having de-aired, waited patiently for the native heart to rest, and added yet more support medications, we tried a third time. On this third attempt, tentatively and gradually, but *successfully*, we weaned the patient from cardiopulmonary bypass. The Novacor artificial heart device was supporting Mr. Kenyon's circulation, and we disconnected the heart-lung machine.

This process may make interesting drama in the later recounting, as here in this chapter, but in real time, it represents the most trying aspect of our cardiac surgical careers. We stare death in the face; usually we win, but not always. It is the "not always" that is foremost in our consciousness as we face the unknown in weaning a critically ill heart—and patient—from the heart-lung machine.

Mr. Kenyon did well afterward, recovering quickly and fully, and embracing life with his artificial heart. Instead of complaining about the noise (a loud, rhythmic thump) or about living with a power cord coming out of his torso, Mr. Kenyon relished his new lease on life—enjoying the fact that he was alive, that he felt well, that he was now safe, and that he could be active again. He made multiple appearances at press conferences and celebrations, in his signature bow tie and suit, always sartorially impeccable. At these events he conducted himself with dignity, intelligence, and articulate, meaningful repartee. His stance, his walk, and his carriage always conveyed a tremendous physical and mental energy and an enthusiasm for life.

The Heart-Lung Machine Requires Anticoagulation (Blood Thinning)

Your blood has, over eons of evolution, been trained to clot if exposed to any surface other than the smooth inner lining of blood vessels (called the endothelium). This is a self-preservation mechanism. If blood cells are encountering a foreign substance, it means that the endothelium has been breached, usually by a traumatic injury. So it is for survival that blood cells exposed to a foreign surface initiate a cascade of events that eventuates in the formation of a clot—to stop the bleeding from the wound that caused the exposure of the blood to external elements. Platelets stick together and bind blood cells in a spiderweb-like meshwork of platelet clumps and strands of proteins.

Now when we place a patient on the heart-lung machine, the blood is exposed to very unnatural foreign surfaces inside the tubing connecting to the machine and within the plastic oxygenator (that percolates oxygen into the tired blood returning from the patient). The blood would clot quite rapidly and extensively—catastrophically—if we did not thin the blood.

For nearly a hundred years, heparin has been used as the anticoagulant of choice. Heparin, in fact, is one of the oldest drugs still in widespread clinical use. Heparin is a naturally occurring substance, and for pharmacologic use, it is concentrated from cow or pig tissues. Heparin is a wonderful drug, reversible instantly by the antidote protamine. But some patients are allergic to heparin, leading to potential extremely serious adverse consequences if it is used.

We have very few suitable alternatives to heparin that can be called upon for use in patients allergic to heparin. We use snake venom or a protein derived originally from bloodsucking leeches. The drug we needed to use in Mr. Kenyon's case is called lepirudin. It has no antidote, so patients continue to bleed even after cardiopulmonary bypass has been terminated. The bleeding finally stops hours later when the body eliminates the lepirudin, largely through the urine.

The Novacor involves a driveline, about the diameter of a pen, which passes out through the abdominal skin. The driveline attaches to a battery pack and computerized controller that are carried on a shoulder strap. The bulky Novacor heart device itself renders quite a noticeable bump in the abdominal contour. With each mechanical beat, the Novacor makes a large noise, like a metal Ping-Pong ball hitting a metal cage. None of this held back or seemed even to bother Mr. Kenyon at any time. He was always chock-full of life. He relished the return of his energy and the renewal of his physical confidence made possible by the Novacor. He viewed himself as well and strong, not sick and dependent as other patients might do and have done.

The artificial heart has become smaller and quieter since that time. For the decade of the 1990s and the early 2000s, the Novacor was like the Chevrolet V-8 of artificial heart devices, a workhorse—reliable and powerful.

Mr. Kenyon did very well, returning to a full family and professional life, as well as becoming a Novacor celebrity of sorts. He could be found visiting the hospital at all hours of the day or night, providing support and education for other heart failure patients facing difficult decisions and interventions. During this time, Mr. Kenyon waited for a suitable human donor heart organ to become available. The Novacor could function only as a "bridge" to eventual heart transplantation.

The only complaint I ever heard Mr. Kenyon voice was that, with the electric power cord, the Novacor prevented him from swimming.

Even a Chevrolet V-8 is not eternal; after 100,000 miles, it can wear out. Mr. Kenyon waited and waited for a suitable donor heart, but none was available. During this time, Mr. Kenyon used his Novacor to the equivalent of 100,000 miles for an automobile engine. Mr. Kenyon's Novacor came to be the longest functioning mechanical heart device in the United States, at nearly 3½ years continuous function. As I said in one of my chart notes, this was, at the time, "one of the longest [artificial heart] durations of implantation in history."

Then came another crisis. We had been monitoring the sound waves put out by the Novacor (with a special listening device on his skin). The engineers at the company knew that eventually the sounds would become abnormal, signaling an impending device malfunction. Please recognize that when the device in question is a mechanical heart, "malfunction" is equivalent to death. This Novacor had given Mr. Kenyon 168,148,000 heartbeats!

Mr. Kenyon's Novacor, at the artificial heart equivalent of 100,000 miles, began to manifest occasional abnormal sound wave signals. We discussed this with Mr. Kenyon. Each time I had a talk with him about this, and the consequent advisability of changing the Novacor preemptively, I could sense the cogs of his spectacularly keen and analytical brain turning. "No thanks," he would tell me. "I will take my chances with the Novacor." Calculating risk is his job—that is where an insurance reinsurer must excel in order to be successful.

We all were very worried about Mr. Kenyon's Novacor. We brought him into the hospital to have him under observation. Of course, in case of catastrophic mechanical failure of the Novacor device, there was not much we could do—even if I was standing at the bedside in his room at that very time. In fact, even with him in the hospital, there was probably nothing that could be done quickly enough to save his life.

Mr. Kenyon took all this remarkably in stride, with an inner and outer peace and calm—and, I daresay, confidence in his decision to "ride it out." He revealed to me at one time that he held out so long because he had figured that, in the winter months in which we found ourselves, car accidents were much more likely. And car accidents are the most common source of heart organs for transplantation. Reader, please do not take this the wrong way. The waiting donor and the transplant team wish no one—NO ONE—ill. But the whole principle of heart transplantation is to take a tragedy and turn it into a miracle. Anyway, Mr. Kenyon figured that, with a bad winter in evidence, it was likely he would get a heart before the Novacor failed.

The renowned heart failure specialist, and an associate dean of our medical school, Dr. Forrester "Woody" Lee, had his own conversations with Mr. Kenyon, encouraging preemptive device replacement, but our patient was steadfast. As time went on, however, his Novacor sound signals became more and more frequently abnormal. The engineers at Novacor called me weekly to be certain that I was aware of this ominous development and that I fully recognized its significance. In equivalent engineering-speak, they were telling me to expect the device to fail suddenly—and soon—leading to Mr. Kenyon's death.

There had been a few close calls for getting a donor heart organ, as on November 26, 2000, and again on June 28 and July 30, 2001, when we actually admitted Mr. Kenyon to the hospital for transplantation. But the preoperative cross-match showed that the immunologic compatibility of recipient and prospective donor was not satisfactory. Mr. Kenyon went home without his organ. This is often a discouraging event for a human being waiting for a life-sustaining heart transplant organ, but Mr. Kenyon's mental fortitude is so great that he never lost his indomitable spirit or optimistic outlook.

We were well into December, and the calls from the Novacor engineers were becoming more and more ominous. On December 31, they called to report that end-stage prefailure signals had been detected. I went to Mr. Kenyon's room, sat on the edge of his bed (as is my wont for intense patient sessions), and had yet another heart-to-heart discussion. "Mr. Kenyon," I said with great respect, "I don't think we can get any more time out of your Novacor. It has done yeoman's work. I think it is about to fail. I think we should replace it."

Now replacing a Novacor is a huge undertaking. There was very little clinical, surgical experience with a replacement operation. There was virtually no experience taking out Novacor devices that had been in place as long as Mr. Kenyon's. Getting through the breastbone and back in to the heart was exceedingly dangerous. The heart scars against the breastbone. So does the outflow tubing from the Novacor, carrying all the patient's bloodstream. Reentry can lead to catastrophic hemorrhage from the heart or the outflow graft—essentially from sawing into the heart or graft. The patient exsanguinates instantly. As well, the abdominal pocket where the huge Novacor device resides commonly scars and contracts tightly against the Novacor itself and its tubes and connectors.

So although I was strongly recommending to Mr. Kenyon that we replace his Novacor, I faced the prospect with some trepidation.

To my surprise, Mr. Kenyon said, "John, let's go ahead. Let's do it right away." His mental calculations had led him to conclude that the risk-benefit ratio of further delay was unfavorable.

My New Year's Eve dance card was now filled. We took Mr. Kenyon to the operating room at about 6 p.m. on New Year's Eve, 2002. We were all so concerned about the potential for catastrophic device failure that we did not wish to wait a single extra minute after Mr. Kenyon gave us the "green light."

Frank Beering, Novacor's chief engineer, came off his Christmas/ New Year's holiday to take the "red-eye" flight back East to be present in the OR for the explant/reimplant. Frank had personally followed the deteriorating sound signals in Mr. Kenyon's aging Novacor device. Frank was exceptionally capable, accessible, and devoted to optimizing patient outcomes.

We had another problem at hand. Mr. Kenyon had become allergic to heparin. Heparin is a powerful blood thinner that is essential for conducting open-heart surgery. Heparin has the wonderful beneficial characteristic that its effects are instantly reversible by another drug, called protamine. So we give heparin just before going onto the heart-lung machine—going "on bypass," so to speak—and we reverse it just after coming off bypass. This management of blood thinning works quite well and underpins the success of open-heart surgery worldwide.

But in light of his heparin allergy, Mr. Kenyon could not be administered this drug. There are no suitable alternatives. To give you an idea, one of the heparin alternatives is snake venom. (We used an alternative, but similarly unpalatable, heparin substitute.) It thins the blood, but it has no antidote. So the patient bleeds and bleeds postoperatively. This is a terrible complication for a reoperative procedure like the one we were about to start on Mr. Kenyon.

We had two bright Greek residents who stayed that night to participate in the operation, Dr. George Tolis (whose dad is an accomplished heart surgeon in his native country) and Dr. Constantine Lovoulos, both of whom have since gone on to distinguish themselves in their own careers.

I was fortunate that my special colleague, Dr. Gary Kopf, a pediatric cardiac specialist, agreed to help and stayed with our team all night. Dr. Kopf may just be the finest human being I have ever met. He is a fantastic surgeon. He is brilliant. But above all, he is a man of the highest moral fiber. He is confident in himself, and he has never succumbed to the machinations and subterfuges that abound in such a competitive field as heart surgery. He knows his own worth and does not need to belittle others or toot his own horn. His only concern is that the patient do well. He has no ego issues or needs. He feels genuinely happy when a colleague does well, and he shares the grief when a colleague has a problem. To my mind, the empathetic characteristic expressed in the last sentence constitutes the very essence of true friendship. I was very fortunate, as was Mr. Kenyon, that Dr. Kopf selflessly gave up his New Year's Eve to perform with us what proved to be an exceptionally difficult operation.

From the moment we first made the incision in Mr. Kenyon's chest that night, we had a tiger by the tail. We could not even get into the chest. The breastbone, as it had healed, had grown completely around the tubes and connectors as well as the body of the Novacor itself. We were dealing with 3½ years of bony scarring. Each time we cut a millimeter, we held our collective breath, as any knife stroke could slice into one of the tubes, leading to instant exsanguination and Mr. Kenyon's death.

We worked for hours and hours, just trying to get a foothold, a single spot where we could make our way into the chest. The scar did not give, and it did not end. I worked and worked. Then Dr. Kopf took the scissors and blade and worked and worked. We each did our best to expose the heart safely and to encourage one another. (Often in cardiac surgery, encouragement of the surgeon across the table can be one of the most important functions of the first assistant—facilitating a difficult or dangerous operation to go forward—like slipping into four-wheel drive when a vehicle is stuck in the snow.) Time and time again, Dr. Kopf and I discussed calling the chest impenetrable, closing up, and turning back.

But instead, we persisted. As I said later in my operative note:

There have been telemetry data indicating impending failure of the device. The number of misfires has accelerated. We have been informed by the Chief Engineer of the manufacturer that a complete device failure is imminent. The patient is brought to the operating room on an urgent basis for device replacement.

This procedure was extremely long and extremely difficult and dangerous. The two surgeons worked for hours to free up the ventricular assist device. The healing bone had grown in and around both the inflow and outflow conduits, and it was extraordinarily difficult to dissect. The conduits were at constant risk during this process of dissection.

The [body's] incorporation of this device was extremely severe, with dense fibrous tissue in addition to the encircling bony tissue.

We had to go on bypass via the large artery and vein in the groin in order to proceed any further. We did so. With the heart-lung machine now managing the circulation, we deliberately cut through the conduits, just to permit access to the bottom of the breastbone.

We were able to gain the needed access in this way. As my notes explain:

A new [Novacor] device was placed. . . . A transition was made from one pump to the other. The heart–lung machine was turned down as the [new] Novacor was turned up. The Novacor functioned well. (It was an identical device to the original, but fresh and new, with "no miles on the clock.")

We were breathing a bit easier, but not easy by any means. Again from my notes:

The patient was quite unstable and it was deemed inappropriate to do further diagnostic or therapeutic measures for this [instability] *at this particular time.*

In other words, it was unclear whether the patient would survive, but there was nothing further that we could do toward the goal of keeping him alive. We had done what we could do.

Continuing in my operative note:

The patient was transferred to the Cardiothoracic Intensive Care Unit in critical condition. Excess drainage [blood] was anticipated because of the prolonged duration of action and lack of antidote for lepirudin. (See the information box.)

We limped back to the ICU, not knowing whether to expect survival or death. The operation had been long and difficult. We had lost quite a bit of blood (transfusing eight units of blood overall). Because of the irreversible anticoagulant, we were still bleeding. Blood pressure was tenuous.

It was New Year's morning, now 2003. I went home to get a few hours' rest. I knew Drs. Tolis and Lovoulos would take impeccable care of Mr. Kenyon.

In a situation like this one, a surgeon never knows what he will face when he returns after a few hours' rest. One may well find a struggling, moribund patient with little chance of survival.

I returned after a few hours to a shock. Wondrously, the bleeding had stopped. The blood pressure had stabilized. Mr. Kenyon was awake and gesturing that he wanted the breathing tube removed.

This was unbelievable. I could never have hoped for such a positive, nearly instantaneous turnaround. I was pleasantly flabbergasted. A feeling of warmth engulfed me, not quite confidence but a sense that we were now wagging the tiger by his tail.

Mr. Kenyon continued to improve hour by hour. Soon, he was extubated and talking as if nothing had happened.

I went home to catch some more shut-eye.

That's when the shocking surprise came.

We had toiled seemingly endlessly to remove and replace a dysfunctional mechanical heart on the verge of catastrophic failure. The patient had made a remarkable, but still very early and tenuous, recovery.

All of this had taken place because no suitable donor heart had become available for 3½ years.

Then I got the call, a real New Year's Day surprise. A HEART WAS AVAILABLE, AND IT WAS A GOOD IMMUNO-LOGIC MATCH. We had waited three and a half long years without a suitable heart. We had changed the Novacor in a nearly undoable, unsurvivable operation just yesterday to prepare for the long-haul wait for an organ. And now, a few hours later, we had a suitable donor heart. Go figure. What are the chances of this? My wife says this was analogous to adopting a baby and then finding out you are pregnant.

Now what do we do? Mr. Kenyon had just come through a tremendous ordeal. It was almost inconceivable to submit him to another operation at this time—less than twenty-four hours after finishing the Novacor exchange. But how could we turn down this potential donor heart—the very first suitable match in ages?

I went and sat again on Mr. Kenyon's bed in the ICU. Re-markably, he was completely awake and lucent and fully able to have a serious, complex conversation. I told him a heart was available. I told him I doubted that a human being could take a transplant operation after what he had just been through. I told him I did not want to lose the donor heart. Every prior heart we had evaluated had been immunologically unsuitable for Mr. Ken-yon. This one was a good match.

He stopped my conversation. "Let's go for it," he said without hesitation. "You'll get me through it." He had pondered briefly, done his actuarial-type calculations, and resolved, without hesitation, to go forward. This man, it seemed, was never uncertain about his decisions—nor was he ever short on courage.

I am sure, reader, that you recognize the tremendous, almost unimaginable, courage reflected in Mr. Kenyon's decision.

Off we went to the operating room. By now, by the time the organ was retrieved, it was January 2, 2003. As I said in my operative note:

The patient is a 62-year-old male with a long history of ischemic cardiomyopathy and LVAD treatment who had his LVAD changed two days previously. He also has a heparin allergy requiring lepirudin treatment. He was quite unstable after the recent LVAD change with significant bleeding. This has resolved. The patient has made an excellent recovery. A donor heart has become available for this patient. The patient has a long history of positive [unfavorable] cross-match to donor hearts. This donor heart was good size with good hemodynamics and normal cross-match. For this reason, we accepted the heart, even at this early date after the recent open-heart surgery for LVAD change.

Dr. Tellides, Dr. Lovoulos, and I headed to the operating room to do a heart transplant. It was another very hard operation. The large, dysfunctional native heart did not wish to exit Mr. Kenyon's body very easily. The lepirudin was again an obstacle. But we persevered.

The new—human—heart was in. It took a tentative beat, then some more, and more and more, and stronger and stronger.

And that heart is still pumping like a champ eleven years later. During those years, Mr. Kenyon has been the most wonderful advocate for heart transplantation. He has counseled many dozens of patients facing similar circumstances, and decisions, to the ones over which he triumphed.

As you know from the introduction to this chapter, Mr. Kenyon returned to competitive swimming as soon as his recovery and his health permitted, first competing in the 2004 U.S. Transplant Games in Minneapolis–Saint Paul, Minnesota. By the time of the 2006 U.S. Transplant Games in Louisville, Kentucky, he was back in good enough shape to win the silver medal in the 400-meter freestyle event and the gold medal (mentioned earlier) in the 200-meter freestyle event, setting a new national Transplant Games record in the latter event for his age group. In 2008, in Pittsburgh, Pennsylvania, less than two weeks shy of his seventieth birthday, Mr. Kenyon won three bronze medals in freestyle events.

Moving up to a new age bracket (70+) in 2010 in Madison, Wisconsin, Mr. Kenyon won gold medals in the 50-, 100-, 200-, and 500-yard freestyle events, setting new U.S. Transplant Games records in the first three events. The following year, 2011, Mr. Kenyon competed with Team USA at the World Transplant Games in Göteborg, Sweden, winning the 50-, 100-, 200-, and 400-meter freestyle events, setting new World Transplant Games records in all four events.

Knowing this exceptional man has impacted me tremendously.

Mr. Kenyon has certainly made great use of his new, strong heart—putting it through its paces. I am certain the reader has recognized the discipline and dedication required to make the athletic accomplishments recounted above a reality.

This is a man who loves life. This is a man who understands risks. This is a brave man who is not afraid to take risks. This is a man who savors every minute, every hour, every day, and every year of life that constitution, resolve, family love, and medicine, technology, and surgery have given him.

I am proud to know this man and to have participated in his care.

I hope your life has been enriched, reader, by hearing all about this courageous man—just as mine has been.

The Technique of Heart Transplantation

The world was electrified on December 3, 1967, when audacious heart surgeon Dr. Christiaan Barnard performed the world's first successful heart transplant on Louis Washkansky, a fifty-three-year-old grocer, in Cape Town, South Africa. The patient lived for a remarkable eighteen days. From that pioneering moment, heart transplantation has grown into a nearly routine procedure, being performed about two thousand times yearly in the United States. I personally have been involved in more than three hundred heart transplant procedures.

Barnard—handsome, irreverent, eloquent, and with an eye for the ladies—became an overnight media sensation, coming to date such celebrity beauties as Gina Lollobrigida, which led *Paris Match* magazine to declare Dr. Barnard "one of the world's four greatest lovers." What the media did not emphasize was that the bold clinical step taken by Barnard in that first operation was based on more than a decade of painstaking laboratory work by Dr. Norman Shumway and Dr. Richard Lower, regarded by many heart surgeons as the real pioneers of heart transplantation.

I believe that both Shumway and his colleague Lower *as well as* Barnard deserve great credit and respect. Lower and Shumway developed the underlying science, and Barnard bravely and expertly took the bold first clinical step. Shumway went on to develop the world's leading heart transplant center at Stanford University over the decades that followed, and he has earned a spot in the pantheon of surgical scientist/clinicians and teachers.

Even today, we apply the very same surgical technique for heart transplantation that was developed by Lower and Shumway. We remove the heart, leaving the edges of the right and left atria. We sew in the new heart with four lines of carefully placed and tightened sutures: one for the left atrium, one for the right atrium, one for the pulmonary artery, and one for the aorta.

In my view, there is another important side to the earth-shattering first heart transplant performed in 1967 by Barnard—a side less appreciated generally than the technical accomplishment. With that one operation, mankind redefined death. Until that point, death was defined as occurring when the heart stopped.

But a heart donor is generally not useful once the heart has stopped, as the heart suffers immediately from deprivation of blood flow. To be useful, the heart still needs to be beating at the time of harvest and the donor needs to have a good pulse and blood pressure. Now a patient with a good pulse and blood pressure would not have been considered dead before Barnard's operation. But, Barnard reasoned, a person's life has no meaning if the brain has died. So Barnard redefined the death of a human being as having occurred once the brain stops functioning.

This definition, forged that momentous day in South Africa, has withstood the test of time. This definition provides a supply of organs from individuals who have suffered brain death (usually by trauma from a car accident or a fall, or from a gunshot wound or a brain hemorrhage). Please do not think this concept hard-hearted. The whole principle of heart transplantation is to take a tragedy (for the donor) and turn it into a miracle (for the recipient).

I had the privilege of having Dr. Barnard provide the keynote address at one of my Yale symposia in 2001. Some of what I am about to relate is based on hearsay—and I hasten to point this out. Other aspects, I witnessed myself.

We had arranged a year before the conference to have Dr. Barnard travel to Yale to give this talk. Hundreds of heart specialists were attending. My secretary, Rhea, had made all the arrangements. We thought it strange that we had not heard recently from Dr. Barnard. We wrote and called but to no avail. We became concerned that he had forgotten our symposium or had changed his mind. Finally, Rhea contacted Dr. Barnard's agent. As it turned out, so we were told, Mrs. Barnard had finally had enough of Dr. Barnard's womanizing (mind you, the man was seventy-eight at that time), and she had kicked him out. He found himself in a wifely imposed exile in Switzerland. So he had been evicted on short notice, leaving in haste without his papers or calendars. The date of our symposium had crept up without Dr. Barnard being aware.

By the time we understood the situation, there was no longer enough time for Dr. Barnard to fly from Switzerland. Rhea hatched a plan to have Dr. Barnard give his talk by satellite—and she made it work. Now in 2001, this all had a high-tech feel to it that is lost in the current era of Skype and instant transcontinental communication. In 2001, we had to make special satellite arrangements. The transmission waxed and waned, and at times the screen was overcome by horizontal wavy lines. Everyone in the audience knew they were witness to a most special event. The use of satellite communication enhanced the aura of excitement.

Dr. Barnard, with great emotion reflected in his voice, recounted the events of that very first transplant—the trepidation, the ethical dilemmas, and the surgical procedure itself. On a lighter note, I hasten to add that, throughout the lecture, Dr. Barnard flirted by long-distance satellite with Rhea, of whom he had become, trans-telephonically, very fond. Now we could see Dr. Barnard, but he could not see us. The audience was amused to note that Rhea, despite being flattered by Dr. Barnard's flirtatious comments in front of hundreds of distinguished attendees, was very clearly well into the third trimester of her first pregnancy. As moderator of the symposium, I was not able to find a subtle way of relaying this to Dr. Barnard, and the flirtation continued, giving credence to Dr. Barnard's inability to control his pursuit of the female sex.

On a serious note, Dr. Barnard had to choke back tears when describing the conclusion of that very first heart transplant operation. In earlier chapters, you have heard me convey the fearful uncertainty that can accompany attempting to wean a patient from the heart-lung machine at the conclusion of open-heart surgery.

"We tried to come off bypass, but to no avail," Dr. Barnard recounted, his voice faltering and tears just visible in his eyes. "My heart sank," he went on. "We added epinephrine and loaded the heart again. Still, the heart manifested only the weakest semblance of a beat. I was devastated. How could this happen? What would this mean for the future of transplantation? I had taken Mr. Wachkansky alive to the operating room. Now, it appeared, I was going to leave him dead on the table. In desperation, we tried a third time. To my shocked amazement, the heart started to beat. In minutes, it had taken over the circulation. The future of heart transplantation had been secured."

This recounting is my paraphrase from memory. But I can tell you, I was hanging on every word and the words, spoken in a quivering whisper, are etched permanently in my mind. I had only two copies of the video of Dr. Barnard's lecture. One was requested by the Smithsonian Institution, as it was one of the very last public addresses Dr. Barnard made before his death in September of that year. My other copy was lost in the fire at our house.

The newspapers said, on September 2, 2001, that Dr. Barnard had died in his hotel room of an asthma attack after a swim at a coastal resort in Paphos, Cyprus. What the papers did not state, but many colleagues said privately, was that they would be surprised had there not been a woman "involved" in some way in the events at that resort. After all, this is the man who said, "I have a woman in my life at all times. I am very much a sex-orientated man . . . I love the divine talent and vigour and lust for life . . ."

In this regard, I call to mind as well a story the *Telegraph* tells of Dr. Barnard from an earlier time: "At the age of 63 his girlfriend was a 22-year-old South African model, Karin Stezkorn; she became his third wife, but that marriage also ended in divorce, when, aged 77, he set out on a Viagra-fuelled affair with another, even younger, girlfriend."

I include for you the news report on Dr. Barnard's autopsy from the *Cyprus Mail*. I am not clear on how a pathologist can detect bronchial spasm on a postmortem examination. In fact, I did not think that was possible. You can judge for yourself. Whatever the cause of death, this man was a true and gifted pioneer, whose name will be forever rightfully remembered in history.

AUTOPSY CONFIRMS ASTHMA KILLED BARNARD
(Archive Article—Wednesday, September 5, 2001)

SOUTH African heart surgeon Christiaan Barnard died after an intense asthma attack, an autopsy confirmed yesterday, not heart failure as initially suspected by health officials.

Pathologist Eleni Antoniou, who conducted the post mortem yesterday, said that Barnard's heart was in excellent condition, rejecting early speculation that Barnard had suffered a fatal heart attack.

She said the cause of death was a bronchial blockage brought on by the attack. Antoniou said she was told that Barnard, who had been suffering from chronic asthma, had had a severe attack on Saturday night and had another attack on Sunday morning, which proved fatal.

She said Barnard had been under medical treatment for his bronchial asthma for several years. His condition worsened due to high temperatures and high levels of humidity, she added.

Barnard's agent Walter Lutschinger said witnesses had told him that Barnard was grappling with an asthma inhaler just before he collapsed.

Barnard, a frequent visitor to Cyprus, arrived last Thursday for a seven-day break ahead of a tour of Germany and the United States where he was to promote his new book, Fifty Ways to a Healthy Heart.

Barnard made medical history in December 1967 with the world's first human heart transplant on 53-year-old grocer,

Louis Washkansky, who lived for another 18 days before dying of pneumonia.

Barnard, who was a regular visitor to Cyprus, was granted Greek citizenship in 1993 for being a well-known philhellene—a distinction that has only been granted to six people worldwide since 1821.

Barnard's funeral will be held in Beaufort West, Cape Town, where he was born.

Copyright © Cyprus Mail 2004

If you are interested in becoming an organ donor, you can contact the United Network for Organ Sharing (UNOS) at http://www.unos.org/.

EPILOGUE

Thank you, reader, for accompanying me to my patients' bedsides, into the operating room, and literally right into their hearts—and ultimately, and intimately, into their lives.

Every one of these ten special patients summoned the great courage required to combat virulent cardiac illness and to submit themselves to complex and high-risk surgical procedures. Facing heart disease and looking death in the eye, they found this courage inside themselves and saw it fanned and fed by love from their families.

In taking this trip with me, you have witnessed a virtual miracle in Mrs. Solomon's survival from an iatrogenic cardiac rupture—a miracle, perhaps reflective of her lifelong dedication to helping other human beings. You have joined me in my brush with greatness and immeasurable talent when I surgically treated the cardiac illnesses of Dave Brubeck, Robert Ludlum, and Wendell Minor. You have met the loving and trusting Mr. Oliva, who was engaged in his own personal battle at the very moment that our country was being attacked on September 11, 2001. You have shared the remarkable story, recounted in her own words, of Carmella, who survived her ruptured aortic dissection, became Patient No. 1 in our aneurysm database, and, via her critical illness, "introduced" me to the remarkable Dr. John Rizzo, who became a superb colleague in our aortic investigations. You have learned of a mother, father, and their young children who were pronounced "dead" after a frigid drowning—yet the youngest child called me out of the blue on the phone twenty years later. You have learned how the death of brave, talented Robert Norton affected me deeply because of the memory of my classmate, who also lost his own life suddenly and prematurely from Marfan's syndrome. You have experienced the passion of NFL Referee Bill Vinovich for his profession and for his family, a passion that motivated him to undergo an especially dangerous and arduous surgical procedure to permit his return to the gridiron. You have watched with me as a keenly intelligent insurance expert put his analytical skills to use in navigating an exceptional maze of challenges—through artificial heart support and ultimately on to cardiac transplantation—permitting him later to win numerous medals at the World Transplant Olympic Games.

Could the rest of us rise to the level of courage, the sheer resolve to live, manifested by each and every one of these courageous patients? Could we stare mortality in the face and back it down?

———

I ask you to think also of how much you have learned, on our journey together, about the heart, its diseases, and how we can repair this so vital but disease-prone organ via dramatic procedures developed and perfected by supremely talented pioneers. You now know about cardiac injuries, coronary artery disease, aortic aneurysms, narrowed heart valves, aortic dissections, and heart failure, transplantation, and artificial hearts, as well as freezing to death and being revived. You have learned so much, but I bet you did not even know it was happening—and you did not need to read a single textbook or take a single test. I hope and expect that the personal drama of each case was the "applesauce" that made the hidden "learning pill" palatable.

Our patients—whom you and I now share—have generously revealed the details of their illnesses, treatments, and lives. But if you think about it, I have bared my soul to you as well. You have been at my side for tremendous triumphs, the highest of highs, but also for the lowest of lows. I have let you into my life, sharing my fears, my hopes, my triumphs, and my failures. You have "heard" me cry. I hope that I have conveyed a sense of how fortunate I feel to have been given the opportunity to care for people's hearts. I hope you have sensed my awe and respect for the elegance and beauty of the human body and especially the human heart.

One of the deepest philosophical questions of all time has to do with why God allows bad things to happen to human beings. I doubt we will ever truly understand this. One widely held opinion is that we see only part of the picture—"as through a glass darkly"—and that the reason for such occurrences will ultimately be made clear to mankind. Another opinion is that if life were eternal and devoid of tribulation, we would not appreciate this gift from our Creator.

But if this book has afforded you any insight, I hope it came from witnessing how fully, strongly, and to the very core the possessors of each of these "Extraordinary Hearts," having come face-to-face with mortality, value life itself and treasure every additional moment of life that their courage combined with medical science have made possible.

Thank you, reader, for joining me on this journey.

John A. Elefteriades, MD

APPENDIX

Note to reader: In addition to the illustrations found in this appendix, the reader can find many additional illustrations, patient photos, and pictures of memorabilia on Dr. Elefteriades's website at JElefteriadesMD.com.

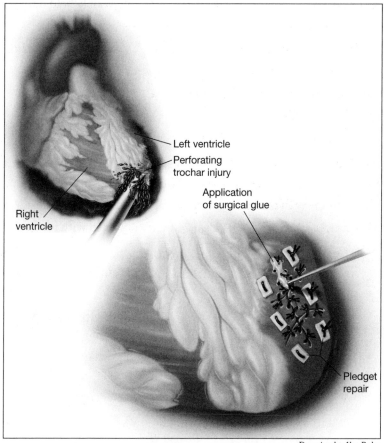

Drawing by Alex Baker

Chapter 1: Mrs. Solomon. Inadvertent trochar perforation of the left ventricle in Emmy case. Note the tip of the trochar tearing through the apex of the heart and the massive bleeding that ensued.

Chapter 2: Dave Brubeck. The coronary arteries, which supply blood to the heart.

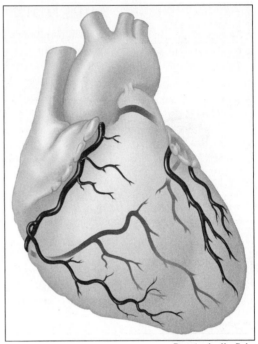

Drawing by Alex Baker

Chapter 2: Dave Brubeck. Arteriosclerosis narrowing a coronary artery. Note the fatty plaque buildup.

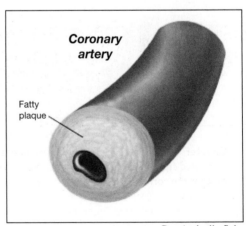

Drawing by Alex Baker

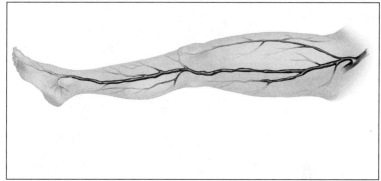

Drawing by Alex Baker

Chapter 2: Dave Brubeck. The saphenous vein, which is used for the coronary artery bypass operation.

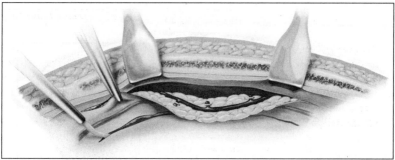

Drawing by Alex Baker

Chapter 2: Dave Brubeck. The internal mammary artery, which is harvested from inside the chest wall. This is the most durable conduit for the coronary artery bypass operation.

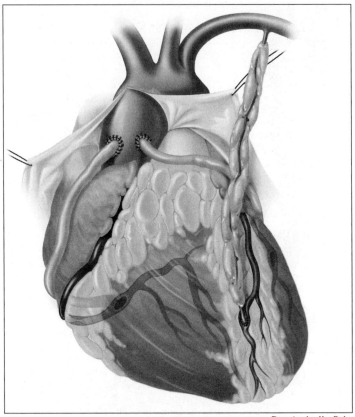

Drawing by Alex Baker

Chapter 2: Dave Brubeck. The completed coronary artery bypass graft operation. Veins are taken from the legs and the mammary artery is harvested from the inside of the chest wall. These are used as conduits for the bypass. We attach each vein to the aorta (to give it a good source of blood flow). We attach the other end of each vein to the coronary artery, beyond the blockage—thus establishing excellent downstream blood supply. The mammary artery already has inflow from its natural origin at the top of the chest, so it only needs one hookup. Each hookup is done delicately, with many microscopic sutures.

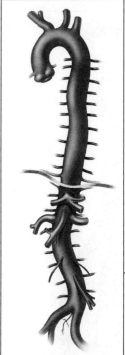

Chapter 3: Mr. Oliva.
Left: A normal aorta. Note normal contour, with "candy cane" shape.

Below: The so-called median sternotomy incision, through the middle of the breastbone, our common "workhorse" incision for cardiac surgery. This incision is actually extremely comfortable postoperatively.

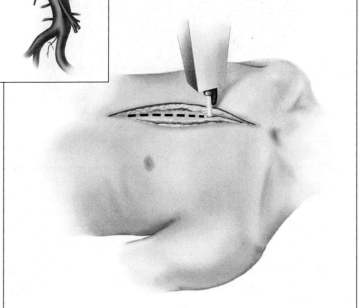

Drawings by Alex Baker

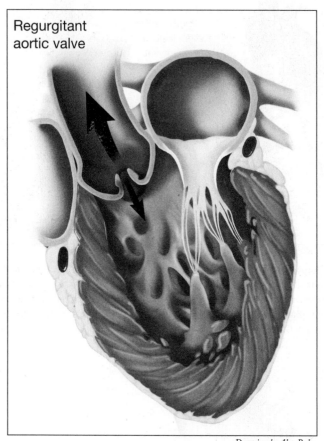

Regurgitant
aortic valve

Drawing by Alex Baker

Chapter 3: Mr. Oliva. Aortic regurgitation, or leakage of the aortic valve. Note the large arrow indicating that most of the blood flow is going appropriately forward through the aortic valve. The smaller arrow shows that some of the blood is inappropriately leaking back through the aortic valve into the left ventricle (pumping chamber).

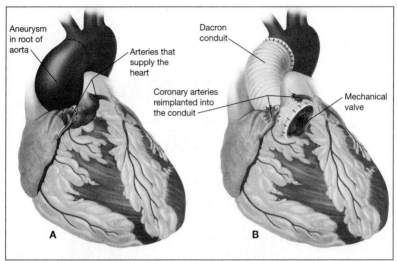

Drawing by Alex Baker

Chapter 3: Mr. Oliva. The operation to replace the aneurismal aortic root. Note how the Dacron conduit, with the built-in mechanical valve, replaces the aortic root. Note that the coronary arteries are reimplanted into the Dacron conduit, a very delicate and exacting connection.

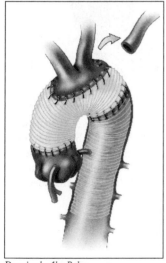

Drawing by Alex Baker

Chapter 3: Mr. Oliva. Replacement of the aortic arch. Note how the arteries to the head and arms are reattached to the top of the arch graft (a serious connection).

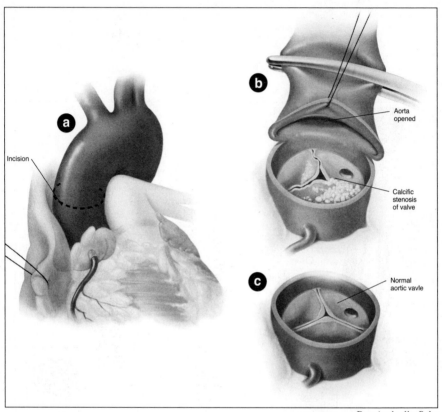

Drawing by Alex Baker

Chapter 4: Robert Ludlum. Aortic stenosis (narrowed aortic valve). (A) shows the incision we make in the aorta to access the valve. (B) shows the calcium deposits, which restrict and narrow the valve. (C) shows how a normal valve should look.

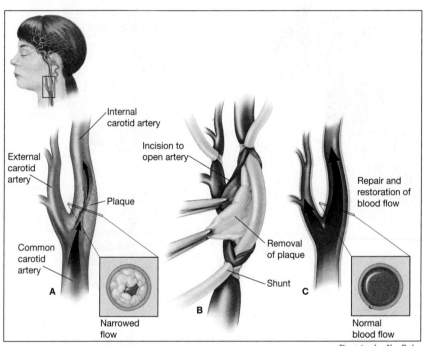

Internal
carotid artery

Incision to
open artery

External
carotid
artery

Plaque

Repair and
restoration of
blood flow

Common
carotid
artery

Removal
of plaque

A

Shunt

B

C

Narrowed
flow

Normal
blood flow

Drawing by Alex Baker

Chapter 4: Robert Ludlum. Carotid stenosis and endarterectomy.
Note the obstructing plaque, and the technique of its removal.

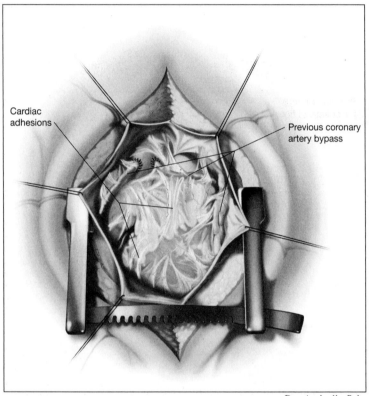

Drawing by Alex Baker

Chapter 4: Robert Ludlum. Cardiac adhesions. Note how the body membranes "stick together" after a first cardiac procedure. This makes reentry for a second procedure difficult and dangerous.

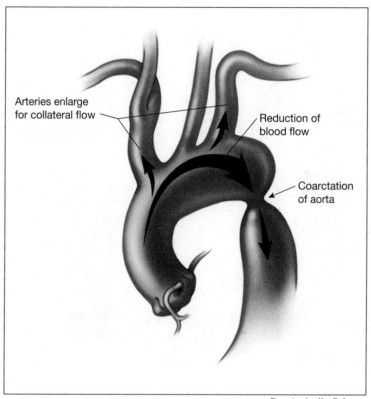

Drawing by Alex Baker

Chapter 6: Wendell Minor. Coarctation of the aorta.

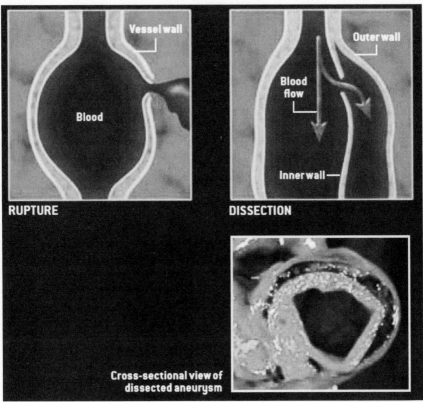

Reproduced with permission from "Beating a Silent Killer,"
J. Elefteriades, Scientific American, *August 2005.*

Chapter 7: Carmella. Schematic depiction of aortic aneurysms. Rupture in upper left. Upper right schematizes aortic dissection; note splitting of aortic wall into two layers, with blood flowing into both channels. Lower right is an actual image, a cross-section, of a dissected aorta; note the "two barrels."

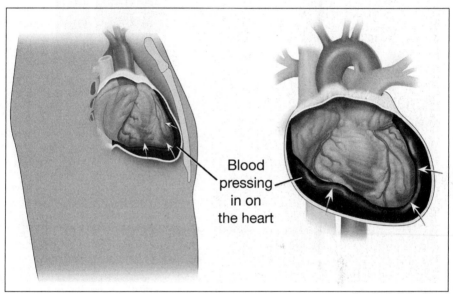

Blood
pressing
in on
the heart

Drawing by Robert Flewell

Chapter 8: Robert Norton. A schematic representation of the physiology of tamponade. In nonmedical jargon, the blood under pressure in the pericardial (heart) sac squeezes the heart shut. Then the heart cannot pump because the heart cannot fill.

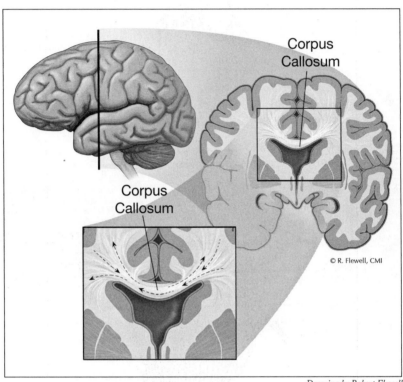

Drawing by Robert Flewell

Chapter 8: Robert Norton. The corpus callosum is the structure deep in the brain that connects the right and left hemispheres of the brain, coordinating the function of the right and left sides.

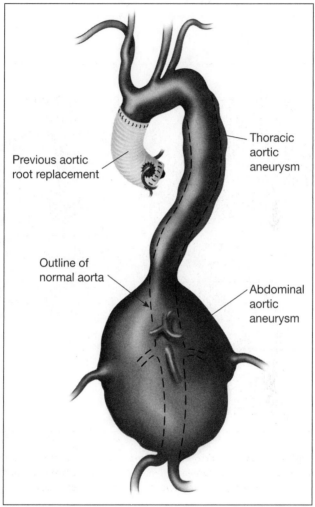

Previous aortic root replacement

Thoracic aortic aneurysm

Outline of normal aorta

Abdominal aortic aneurysm

Drawing by Alex Baker

Chapter 8: Robert Norton. This schematic shows a huge thoracoabdominal (chest and belly) aortic aneurysm, replicating Robert Norton's.

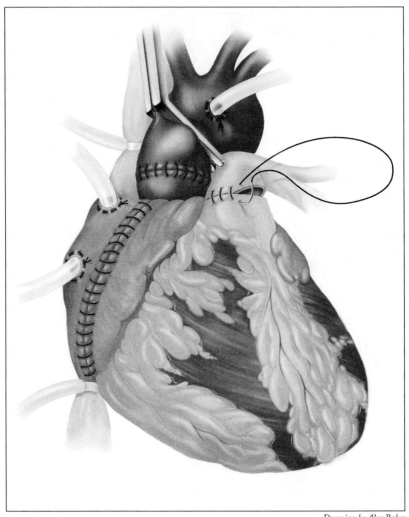

Drawing by Alex Baker

Chapter 10: Pete Kenyon. The procedure of cardiac transplantation.
Note suture lines.